Tips and Tricks Series
The Neck
by

Jane Johnson

D1826347

This book is a privately printed copy.

About the *Tips & Tricks Series* for Therapists
This is a series of books designed to support and
inspire massage therapists and students of
physiotherapy, osteopathy and sports therapy. Each
book contains three parts: assessment tips,
treatment tips and aftercare tips. Readers are
encouraged to contact the author with comments
and suggestions. Let's share our knowledge and
skills to help develop competent and confident
therapists worldwide.

Other titles in the *Tips & Tricks for Therapists*
series:
The Knee
The Thorax
The Lumbar Spine
The Shoulder

TIPS & TRICKS SERIES

THE NECK

Jane Johnson

Privately printed copy, 2013

Designed by Lee Lawrence
Illustrations by Jair Herculano and Graham
Rosewarne
Edited by Margaret Doyle, Ruth Midgley,
Karalynn Thomson

Printed and bound in the UK by PublishPoint,
from KnowledgePoint Limited, Reading

ISBN: 978-0-9927517-0-8

First published in 2013 by Jane Johnson

For information contact:

Jane Johnson
Jane@janejohnson.co.uk

INTRODUCTION

This is the first book in the *Tips & Tricks for Therapists* series. It is the first book in the series because the neck is that part of the body many therapists admit they are sometimes scared to treat. The neck is crammed with nerves, and we are rightfully taught to take care when working on this region of the spine, but to such an extent that some therapists become anxious about treating it with anything other than very general, gentle massage.

Of course, gentle massage involving effleurage and petrissage is all that is sometimes required. But often the relief provided is short term, the client's problem persists, or you feel 'stuck' as to what advice you can give your client to help them self-manage their problem. This book provides you with ideas for the assessment, treatment and aftercare of those clients who come to you complaining of problems such as general neck pain or stiffness, the kinds of clients so many of us come across on a regular basis.

If you have ever felt uncertain about how to treat this part of the body, and your skills and confidence need a boost, then this book is for you.

6   The tips and tricks provided here are effective and safe. They fall within the remit of qualified therapists. If you are a newly qualified therapist, or have not practiced for some time, the information you find here will improve your understanding and will help you to gain confidence. If you are an experienced therapist, I hope you too will find something useful among these tips.

If you know of a useful tip that you think should be included in the next edition of the book, please let me know and I will consider using it with your permission.

I also welcome comments and suggestions.

You can contact me at jane@janejohnson.co.uk.

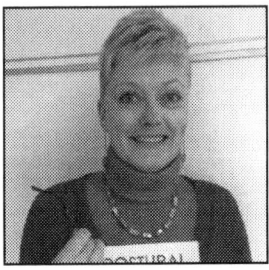

All the titles in the *Tips & Tricks* series assume that you have consulted your client and taken a general medical history. You have decided that your client is safe to be assessed and treated and they have given consent for this.

Each of the three sections of this book contains a list of tips. Within these, embedded in the text, you will find additional tips marked in *italics*.

You will also find common questions boxed and italicized.

CONTENTS

Part 2 Neck Treatment *Tips & Tricks*

Part 3 Neck Aftercare *Tips & Tricks*

Part I Neck Assessment
Tips & Tricks

In this part of the book you will find lots of *tips* on how to assess someone who comes to you with a neck complaint. This might be something as simple as a stiff neck, a sore neck, someone who feels tense after sitting for long periods of time at work, or perhaps even someone who had an injury many years ago but still gets the odd 'niggle' in their neck. It could be someone you have been treating for many months, or it could be a new client.

The *tips and tricks* you will find here are not arranged in any particular order. The information here is not designed to replace any training you have had. Instead, it is designed to support and enhance your existing skills and is crammed with the kinds of *tips* you may not have come across, *tips and tricks* I have picked up over the years and which I hope you too will find beneficial in your practice. Of course, there will be material with which you are familiar, but I am hoping that you will discover a selection of assessment tips which make you think, "Ah, I haven't tried that, maybe that will work!"

Most therapists reading this book will be sensible enough to know that you would not carry out any of these assessments on a person with an acute injury to their neck, such as whiplash. You will find only a few *cautions* written into the text in this part of the book, and the reason is that the majority of these assessments are perfectly safe for the majority of people you are likely to be assessing. Where *special caution* is needed, this has been stated, so please read the whole tip before attempting the assessment.

TIP 1 ASSESSING RANGE OF MOVEMENT (ROM)

When a client comes to you with a neck problem, one of the simplest assessments you can do—once you have finished asking questions—is to observe which movements they can (and can't) perform with their neck. You may already be doing this and may know that this is called a Range of Movement (ROM) test. Because you are going to ask the client to perform the movements themselves, this is an *active* ROM test. You may have heard of passive ROM tests, where the therapist takes a joint through its range of movement, but in this book, for this part of the body, we are only going to do active ROM tests.

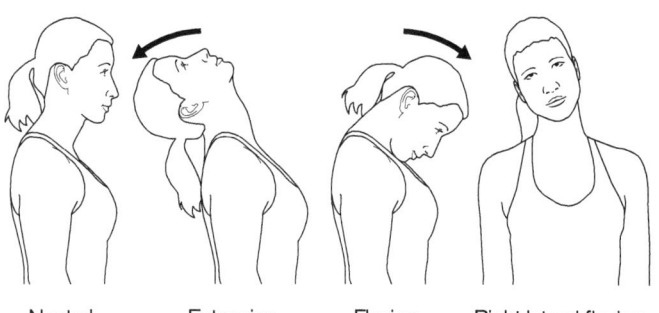

Neutral   Extension   Flexion   Right lateral flexion

The neck can move in six ranges for the purposes of this assessment: flexion/extension, right lateral flexion/left lateral flexion and right rotation/left rotation.

A good place to start when assessing the neck is to demonstrate to your client what it is you want them to do, and then to watch how they perform the movements and to note what they say.

Question: Does it matter which movement the client performs first?

No. If you are new to this form of assessment, one tip is always to perform the movements in the same order, with every client. For example, flexion then extension and back to neutral; right rotation then left rotation and back to neutral; right lateral

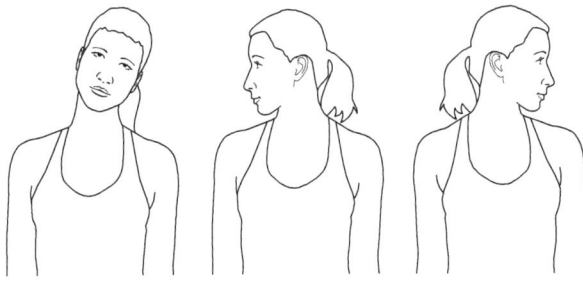

Left lateral flexion   Right rotation   Left rotation

flexion then left lateral flexion, and back to neutral. That way, you are unlikely to miss anything. However, there may be times when you need to make an exception. For example, if a client has already told you that they experience discomfort on a particular movement—rotation of their head to the right, for example—it is sometimes a good idea to ask them to perform this particular movement *last*. The reason for this is that if the client experiences discomfort at the start of the assessment, they may be less willing to continue and you may not discover which movements they can and can't do. So, if a client tells you that they experience discomfort on looking over their right shoulder when trying to reverse their car, make right rotation the last range of movement that you test, checking the other five movements first.

A *tip* here is to make sure that your client does not move their shoulders when performing ROM tests. Clients with neck pain or a stiff neck have a tendency to twist at the waist and move their thorax in order to rotate to the right or to the left, instead of rotating their neck. Similarly, when asked to perform lateral flexion, they have a tendency to raise their shoulders: if lateral flexion to the right is uncomfortable or difficult, they raise their left shoulder, thus appearing to be able to move in this direction when in fact the movement is generated from their torso. Check for these 'cheating' movements by paying close attention to your client's shoulders during the test. If you see movement in the shoulders, instruct your client to start again, whilst keeping their shoulders stationary. By asking the client to keep their shoulders stationary the limitations in their cervical ROM become more apparent and you therefore get a more accurate picture of what they can and can't do with their neck.

Question: Does it matter where you stand when carrying out this assessment?

Some therapists stand behind their clients when assessing active cervical ROM. The advantage is that the therapist can observe the cervical spine. The disadvantage is that the client may feel anxious having someone stand behind them, even though the cervical ROM test is quick to perform: as you know, people are protective of their necks, more so if they are in pain or have suffered with neck problems in the past. Standing in front of your client, you have the advantage of being able to observe their facial expressions. This position is also more conducive to the development of rapport.

18

Question: Are active ROM tests safe for all clients?

Active ROM tests are safe for most people because everyone moves their head through these ranges— and combinations of these ranges—during the day. Active ROM tests may *not* be safe in certain very specific circumstances: following an accident or following surgery to the neck, for example. This book is not designed to help you assess people with cervical trauma. Also, there may be a small group of people for whom caution is needed when asking them to perform active movements involving the head and neck. For example, active ROM tests should be performed with caution if, when taking the client's medical history, you discover your subject suffers from an inner ear disorder such as Ménière's disease. Another example is if they report experiencing dizziness when they look up to the ceiling.

Question: When caution is needed, what instructions might you give the client prior to them performing the test?

Instruct them to move their head *slowly*, or to stop if they feel in any way dizzy or unwell.

TIP 2 HOW TO TELL WHAT'S A 'NORMAL' ROM

So you've tested your client's active cervical ROM. As they were performing the movements you found yourself asking, "How do I know what's a 'normal' range of movement in the neck?" Well, there are many books in which normal ranges of movement can be found. One such is *The Clinical Measurement of Joint Motion* (1994) by the American Academy of Orthopaedic Surgeons. This has clear illustrations and focuses only on this topic so is easy to follow.

However, a good *tip* is simply to assess a lot of people. By doing this you will soon get to build up a kind of visual database, a set of images in your mind as to what's normal and what's not. When you see someone who can only flex their head to the side a little, you will know that they have a ROM *less than* the norm. Conversely, when a client effortlessly bends their head to the side so that their ear appears to almost touch their shoulder, you'll know that they have a ROM *greater* than the norm.

Green, W.B. and Heckman J. D., eds., 1993. *The Clinical Measurement of Joint Motion*. Rosemont, IL: American Academy of Orthopaedic Surgeons.

NORMAL RANGE OF MOVEMENT

Range of Movement	Neutral position	Example
Flexion This could be measured in 0 to 90 degrees from the neutral position. Norm = about 38 degrees Or, it could be measured crudely in terms of how many centimeters (or inches) the subject's chin is from their sternum.	 0°	This person has about 45 degrees of flexion. Their chin is less than 1cm from their sternum. They would appear to have a greater degree of cervical flexion than most people. 45°
Extension This could be measured in 0 to 90 degrees from the neutral position. Norm = about 38 degrees Or, it could be measured crudely in terms of how many centimeters (or inches) the subject's chin is from their sternum.	 0°	This person has about 30 degrees of extension. Their chin is about 22.5cm from their chest. This appears to be slightly less than a normal range. 0°/30°

NORMAL RANGE OF MOVEMENT

Range of Movement	Neutral position	Example
Lateral flexion This could be measured in 0 to 90 degrees from the neutral position. Norm = about 43 degrees Or, you could measure crudely how far the client's ear is from their shoulder.		 In this example our subject has about 22 degrees of left lateral flexion, less than the norm.
Rotation This could be measured in 0 to 90 degrees from the neutral position. Norm = about 45 degrees		

Use the table opposite to help you record five neck assessments. The illustrations at the top of the table are a reminder of the six movements you need to check. One assessment has been filled in for you, for a subject called Mrs Brown, aged 64. From the table you can see that she has 30 degrees of flexion and 20 degrees of extension, 30 degrees of right rotation and 25 degrees of left rotation; 10 degrees of right lateral flexion and 20 degrees of left lateral flexion.

Here is a another *tip:* Assess ten people who drive for a living or who do a *lot* of driving. Assess ten people who are over the age of 70. Assess ten people who have sustained a whiplash injury in the past five years (providing they are safe to be assessed now, of course). Assess ten people who maintain a static posture for long periods of time. Assess ten people who regularly perform yoga. These are arbitrary selections but you get the idea. By assessing similar groups of people, you will soon discover interesting similarities among clients. For example, if you have not done so already, you may discover that, as we age, the range through which we can actively move our neck decreases. Also, movement decreases in one or more ranges following injury if the client has not been properly rehabilitated; and people who regularly perform yoga may have an increase in cervical range, or may maintain their cervical range for longer as they age.

Subject	Flexion	Extension	Right rotation	Left Rotation	Right lateral flexion	Left lateral flexion
Mrs Brown Aged 64	30	20	30	25	10	20

It would be wrong to say that all elderly people have a reduced range of movement in their neck. Some may have an increase in range—maybe they are fitness enthusiasts and include neck stretches in their routines, or perhaps they had increased mobility to start with. You get the idea. So, whilst we do not want to pigeonhole people, the more people you assess, the more likely you are to be able to identify when a client has a ROM that is greater or less than normal, taking into account their age, occupation, lifestyle and health factors.

The problem with measuring ROM is that people's necks can 'hinge' in different places. That is, some of the vertebrae can remain 'stuck' whilst others move more freely, so the movement we observe is not coming equally from each of the seven cervical vertebrae. Vertebrae do not form hinge joints, as you know, but the movement impairment that is sometimes observed when people perform ROM assessments may be thought of as a hinging *movement*.

Question: What if a client reports a problem involving movement, yet when you test them, they appear to have a normal ROM? That is, flexion, extension, lateral flexion (both left and right) and rotation (both left and right) all appear fine, with little or minimal discomfort.

There are many factors contributing to neck discomfort (movement is *one* of them). The thing to remember is that in daily life we *combine* these movements. For example, if you are holding this text slightly lower than horizontal in order to read it, your neck may be a little flexed. If you were to keep your neck flexed but look over your right shoulder, you are now combining forward flexion with right rotation. Similarly, if you look up into the sky and trace the path of an aircraft as it passes overhead, your neck is in extension and will involve a degree of rotation, depending on which way the aircraft is moving. Try rubbing your left ear on your left shoulder by moving your head. You are now combining left lateral flexion with both right and left rotation. So, it may be that a client's condition is aggravated not by one movement, but by a combination of movements, and this is worth remembering as it provides further clues that will help you determine what the problem, and the appropriate treatment, might be.

TIP 3 USING A GONIOMETER TO MEASURE CERVICAL ROM

If you want to be more accurate in your cervical ROM measurement you could use a goniometer. Begin with your client seated, preferably with their back supported and feet flat on the floor. Then, position your goniometer as shown in this tip and measure the different ranges. Follow the instructions provided on the following pages to help you to measure flexion, extension, lateral flexion and rotation.

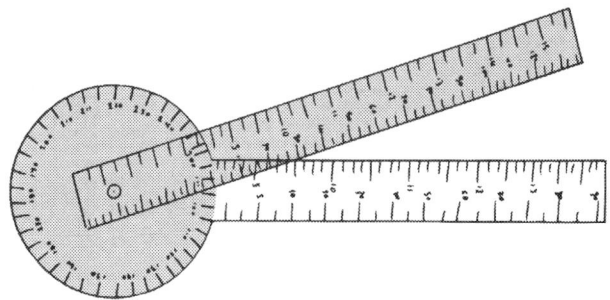

Questions to ask yourself:

How easy did I find using a goniometer to measure cervical ROM?

Did I find any particular aspects easier than others? For example, was it easier for me to measure rotation than lateral flexion?

What could I do differently next time to improve my skill in using a goniometer to measure cervical ROM?

Would using a larger or smaller goniometer help?

Was the client positioned correctly? Could I change the position in any way to make measuring easier or more accurate?

How good was I at giving instructions to my subject? Did they understand? Is there anything I need to do differently next time?

How easy was it for me to record my findings?

Questions to ask about your client:

How do their ROM measurements compare with other subjects of their age and gender?

Are there differences in left- and right-sided readings?

Have these measurements changed over time and if so, in what way?

In what way might a ROM finding relate to my client's daily life - does decreased (or increased) ROM make any daily tasks more difficult?

Would helping to alter ROM improve my client's quality of life in any way? For example, if they had greater cervical rotation would that help when they are looking over their shoulder to reverse their car?

How might I explain ROM findings to my client in a way that is reassuring?

Measuring neck flexion with a goniometer

1. Position the center of your goniometer over the external auditory meatus.

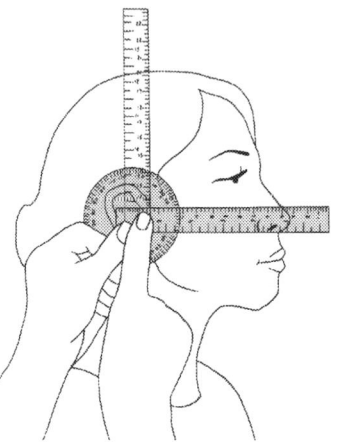

2. Ensure that the arm of the goniometer that is to be stationary is perpendicular to the floor.

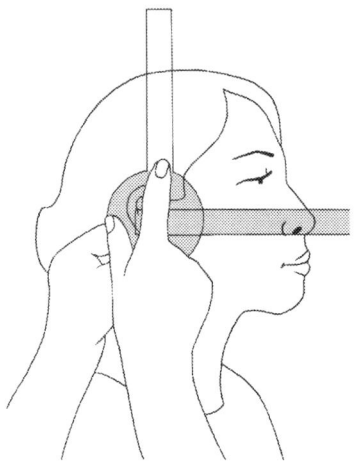

3. Align the arm of the goniometer that is to move with nares.

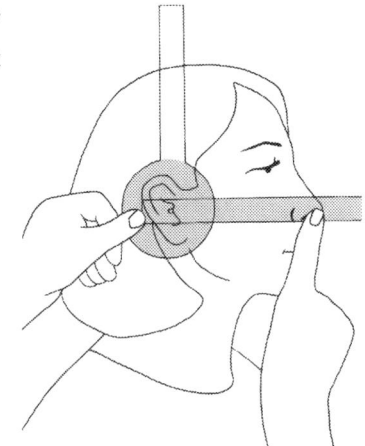

4. Ask your client to take their chin as close to their chest as possible and, as they do this, move the arm of the goniometer to keep it aligned with nares. Be sure to keep the stationary arm of the goniometer fixed. Take your measurement.

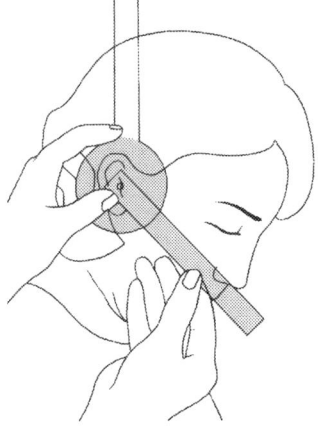

Measuring neck extension with a goniometer

1. Position the center of your goniometer over the external auditory meatus.

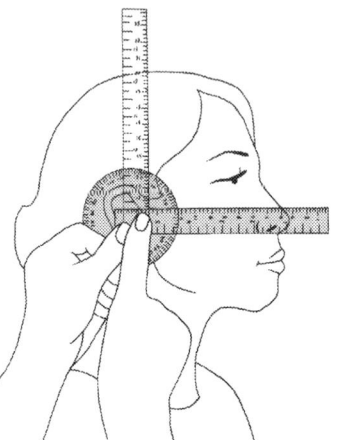

2. Ensure that the arm of the goniometer that is to be stationary is perpendicular to the floor.

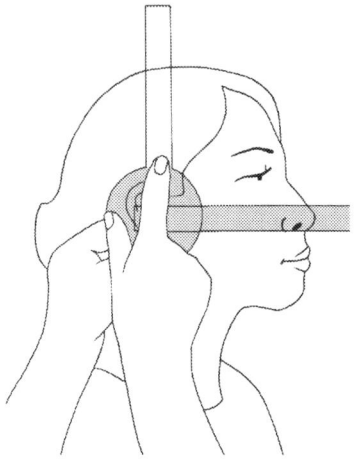

3. Align the arm of the goniometer that is to move with nares.

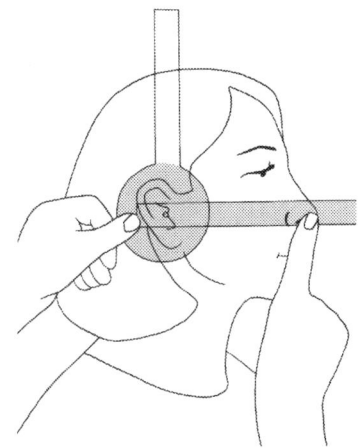

4. Ask your client to take their head as far back as possible, trying to get the back of their head to touch the top of their back. As the client does this, move the arm of the goniometer you have aligned with nares. Be sure to keep the stationary arm of the goniometer fixed. Take your measurement.

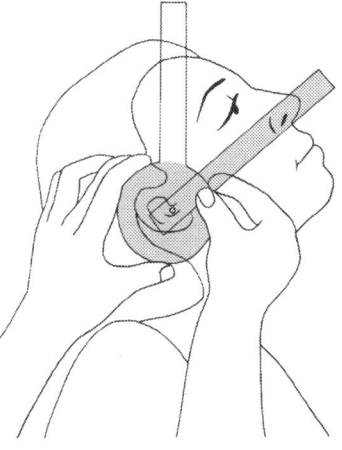

Measuring lateral flexion of the neck with a goniometer

1. Locate the spinous process of C7.

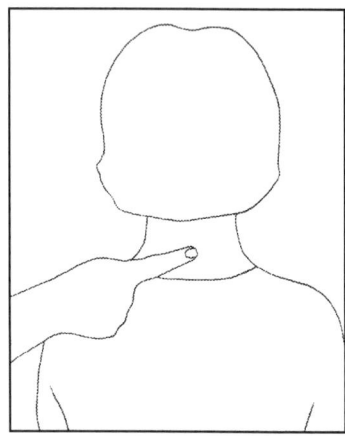

2. Locate the occipital protuberance and spinous processes of thoracic vertebrae.

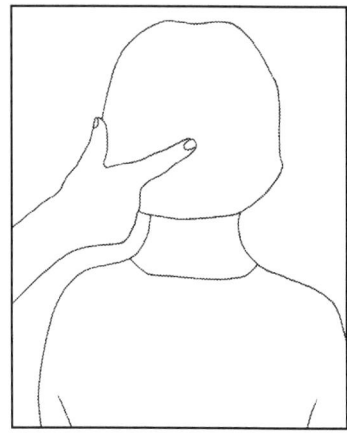

3. Position the center of your goniometer over C7, with the stationary arm over the spinous processes of thoracic vertebrae and the moveable arm over the occipital protuberance.

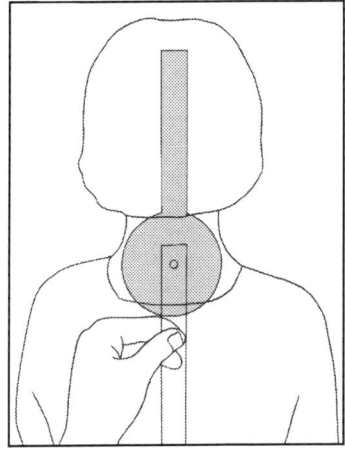

4. Instruct your client to keep their shoulders still and down as they move their head to try and get their ear to touch the shoulder on that side. Keep the moving arm in alignment with the occipital protuberance and take your measurement at the end of range. Repeat this on the opposite side.

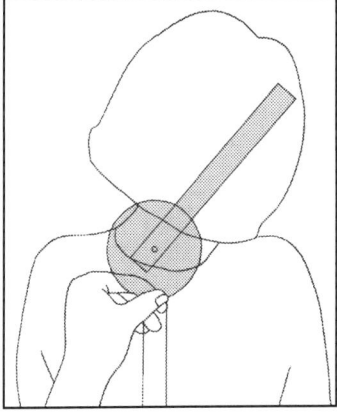

Alternative method of measuring lateral flexion
Lateral flexion can also be measured using a
goniometer as the therapist stands in front of the
client.

1. Start by asking your subject to hold a tongue
depressor between their teeth. These are
inexpensive and maybe obtained from
many pharmacies.

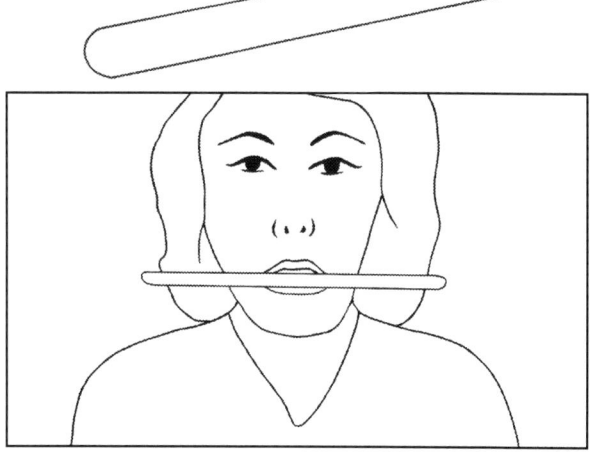

2. Position the goniometer parallel to the tongue
depressor.
3. Ask your client to take their ear to their
shoulder on the side at which you are holding the
goniometer. Move the goniometer as they do this,

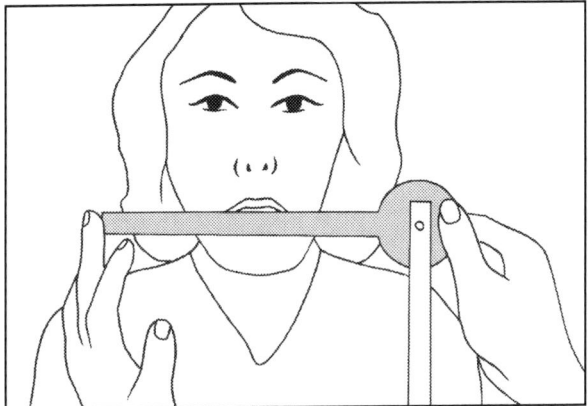

keeping it parallel with the tongue depressor.
Measure the number of degrees of lateral flexion
when they reach the end of their active range of
movement.

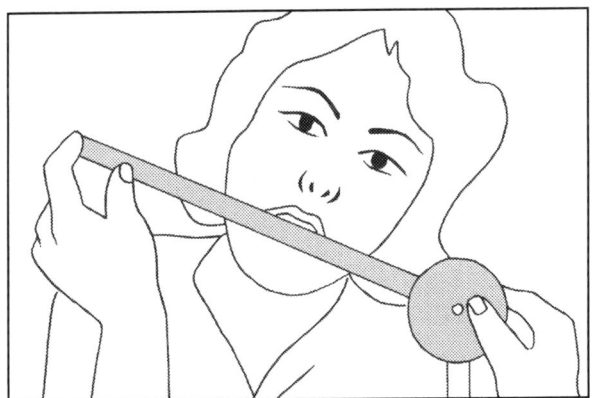

Measuring neck rotation with a goniometer

1. Locate the very top of the head and the acromion process.

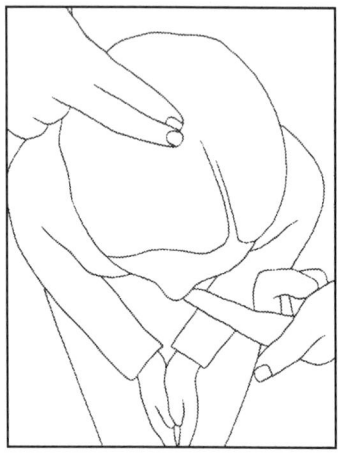

2. Position the center of your goniometer over the center of the head and the stationary arm over the acromion process. Position the moving arm of your goniometer over the tip of the nose.

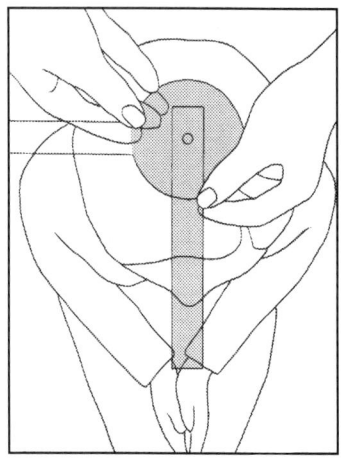

3. Ask your client to try and keep their chest and shoulder still as they turn their head to look over one shoulder. Move the stationary arm of the goniometer as they do this, keeping it aligned with the nose. At the end of range take your measurement. Repeat on the other side.

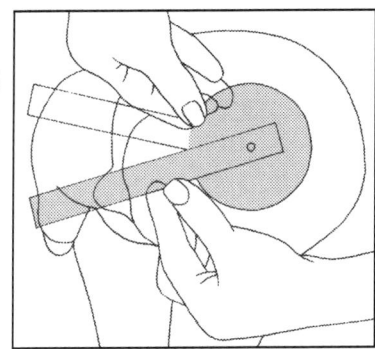

Document your findings
Note the date
Note the position of your client during the ROM tests
Note what equipment you used
Record your measurements
  For example
    flexion 50%
    extension 10%
    right rotation 20%
    left rotation 30%
    right lateral flexion 25%
    left lateral flexion 30%

Record anything else you think was significant.
  For example, 'client was unable to rotate to the right without shrugging right shoulder'.

TIP 4 USING A TAPE MEASURE TO MEASURE CERVICAL ROM

Flexion
Measure the
distance from the
chin to the
sternal notch.

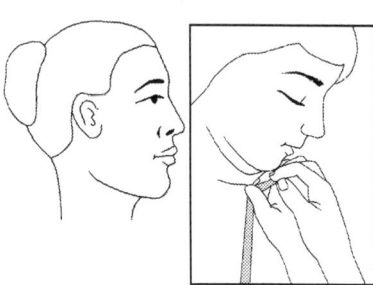

Extension
Measure the
distance from the
chin to the
sternal notch.

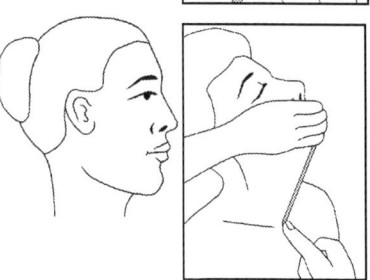

Lateral flexion
Measure the
distance from the
mastoid process
to the acromion
process

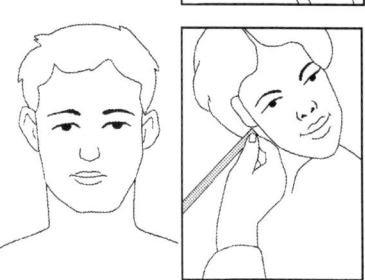

Rotation

Place a mark on your client's acromion process. Measure the distance from the tip of the chin to the acromion process (on the side to which the client rotates).

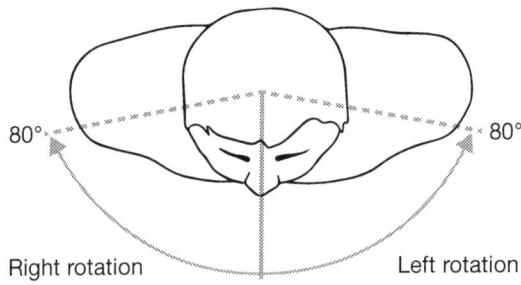

80°   80°

Right rotation   Left rotation

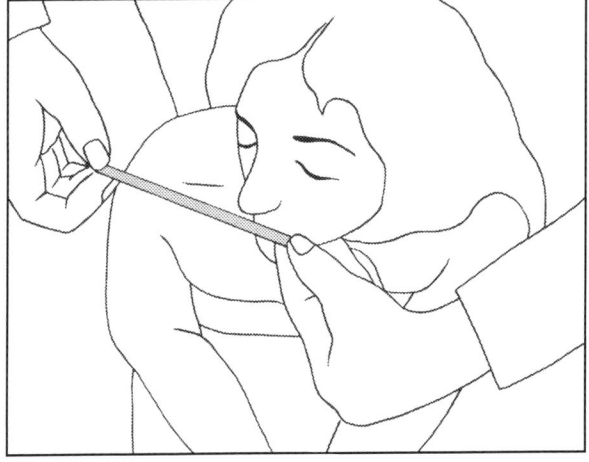

TIP 5 DOCUMENTING YOUR ROM FINDINGS

Let's take the example of a client who comes to you with a stiff neck. You assess them, asking them to do the active ROM test, and then you decide on an appropriate treatment. Assuming that the goal of your treatment is to decrease their feelings of stiffness and/or increase their actual active movement, you will need to document the client's current limitation in ROM, as well as their post-treatment increase in ROM. Here are some ideas.

a) One way to do this is to make a little sketch. It could be a small oval to represent a head, like the cartoons shown here.

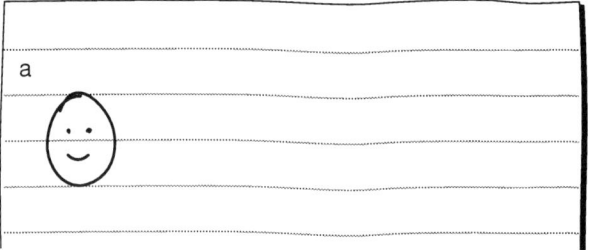

b) Or, it could be a line, either superimposed over
   the sketch or simply on its own.

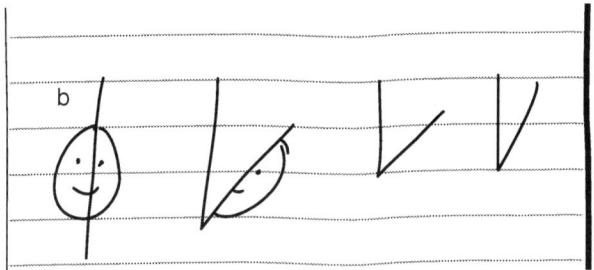

c) Or, you could guestimate in degrees the amount
   by which the range is decreased. For example, if
   rotation was decreased by what you thought was
   five degrees you could write -5° with a line
   representing rotation.

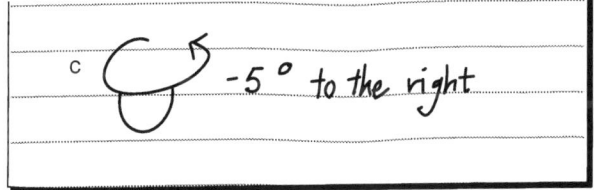

Experiment with different ways to document ROM
findings until you find those that you are
comfortable with and, importantly, which you
will understand when you refer to your notes in
the future.

TIP 6 CHECKING QUALITY OF MOVEMENT

Sometimes a client is able to perform full ROM yet the quality of their movement is poor. Maybe they wince or grimace as they perform the movement (another good reason to face your client when you carry out ROM tests) and yet are still able to perform it fully. Maybe they stop and start, taking their neck through its full range but with hesitancy. Or perhaps you simply get a sense of their caution, that they are guarding themselves. Hesitancy may be common following whiplash injuries, for example, when the tissues are healed but the client is fearful of reinjury. A client with an inability to perform active cervical ROM fluidly could be described as having a 'poverty' of movement. It is as important to document the quality with which a movement may be performed as it is to document the range of movement attained, as this provides yet another piece of your assessment puzzle.

As with your documentation of the actual range of movement, you will need to find a way to record the quality of movement in a way that you understand. 'Poverty', 'hesitancy', 'guarding?', etc. could be useful. Notice that there is a question mark after 'guarding'. This is deliberate because we cannot know as a therapist whether someone is guarding themselves when they move their neck, as this is a subjective assessment of the movement we have observed.

Question: What might you record if you observe a client to have full range of active neck movement yet in order to perform the movements the client keeps wincing?

In documenting *your* observations, would it be appropriate to write something like:

full movement—?pain

What do you think?

TIP 7 DOCUMENTING DISCOMFORT

Many clients visit a therapist hoping to get relief from discomfort in their neck. If you are reading this as an experienced therapist you will know that the words clients use to describe how they are feeling do not always involve the word 'pain'. Have you ever come across someone who says that their neck is 'pulling', 'tight', or that it 'clicks'? Or someone who says they have a 'sore' neck or that it is 'a bit crunchy'? Can you remember whether you repeated the words used by the client, or whether, in response, you said something like, 'so where abouts is the pain?' It can be a challenge to avoid using the word 'pain'. It's a word bandied about, used to embrace a plethora of descriptive terms such as those listed above as well as 'stiff', 'aching' and 'hurt'. But why should it matter? Why not document your client's problem using the word 'pain' as a generally descriptive term? Accurate documentation is important for several reasons. First, because if we use a patient's description of their symptoms as a baseline measurement against which we judge the effectiveness of our treatment, then it's important we do this accurately. 'Pulling' or 'crunching', for example, are descriptions of sensations which we are likely to want to lessen. If, following the treatment of a client with such symptoms, we ask them, "Has your pain diminished?" the answer will be meaningless. What we need to be asking is whether their 'pulling' or 'crunching' sensation has diminished.

Another important reason for using and documenting what clients say is that by doing so people feel that they are being 'heard'. This alone increases the chances of building rapport between the client and the clinician. A third reason for accurate recording of terms used is that this prevents the assessment water from getting muddied. If you start using the word 'pain' too often to describe a client's symptoms, sooner or later the client will start to use the word. This can lead to misdiagnosis and inappropriate treatment.

A final important reason for using the patient's exact terminology is that people tend to use similar words to describe similar diseases, and so having precise words can help with a more precise diagnosis. For example, and very generally, clients experiencing problems involving nerves might describe their symptoms as 'sharp', 'shooting' or 'tingling', whereas those clients suffering bone or muscle problems might use words such as 'deep', 'boring' or 'aching'. Some of the words clients use to describe neck symptoms following whiplash can be very strange indeed, and it is important that as therapists we document whatever words our clients use in order to add to the collective understanding of how such conditions present in the clinical population. This concept is explored in depth in *Pain: the Science of Suffering* by Patrick Wall.

A *tip* for helping you to avoid prompting your clients with use of the word 'pain' is to write out some alternative questions. For example:
"Can you elaborate?"
"What sort of discomfort is it?"
"When did you first notice it?" (rather than "When did you first get the pain?")
"When you say it's uncomfortable, can you be more specific?"

Using these kinds of open-ended questions encourages the client to search for words that best describe their symptoms and can help you discover more about the nature of the problem.

Wall, P., 1999. *Pain: The Science of Suffering*. London: Weidenfeld & Nicolson.

TIP 8 A DIFFERENTIATION TEST

This next test is simple and rather crude but may help determine whether a neck problem is purely muscular, or whether there is an underlying skeletal/ligamentous component. It is a useful test because if you suspect that a client's problem may be due to the cervical vertebrae themselves, or to the ligaments of these joints, it means that you are in a good position to refer your client to a physiotherapist, osteopath or chiropractor for further investigation if the specific assessment of joints is outside your professional remit.

For this test you will need to stand behind your client which, as was noted in *Tip 1* (p.17), has certain disadvantages. However, it is necessary for this particular test. This test relies on what your client says, so it is important to listen to the descriptive terms they use.

First, with your client seated, test their range of cervical movement (ROM) by asking them to perform the movements of flexion, extension, lateral flexion and rotation described in *Tip 1* (pp.14-16). Observe the degree and quality of movement, and ask how the movements feel.

Document these findings. Remember from *Tip 7* (p. 44) to identify the exact words the client uses to describe any discomfort, words such as 'pulling', 'pinching', 'sticking', 'catching' or 'squashing'.

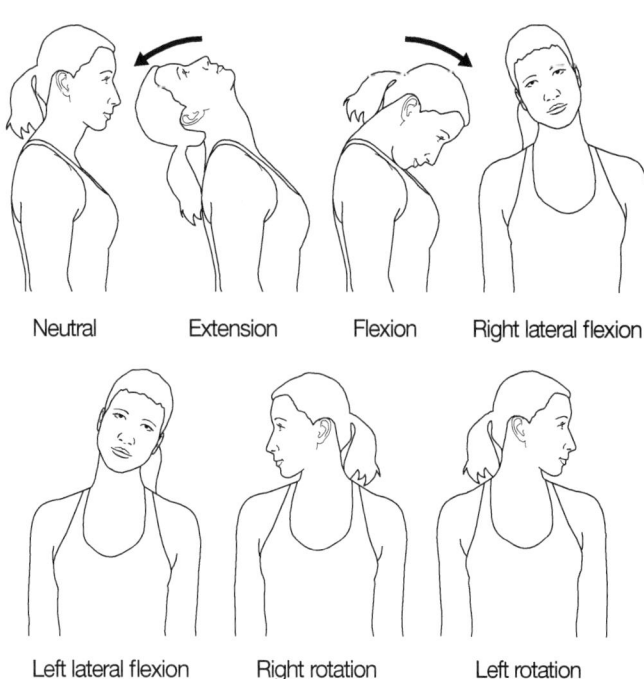

Neutral   Extension   Flexion   Right lateral flexion

Left lateral flexion   Right rotation   Left rotation

Second, still standing behind your seated subject, passively elevate their shoulders, supporting them under the elbow. Safeguard your own posture as you do this to avoid straining your back. Maintaining this position of passively elevated shoulders, ask your client to repeat the active cervical ROM, observe their movements and again get feedback.

Passively elevating the shoulders takes some tension out of the muscles spanning the shoulder-neck region and reduces the pull on their connecting fascia. Therefore, if with passive elevation of the shoulders pain/stiffness/discomfort is *reduced*, and ROM is *increased*, there is a

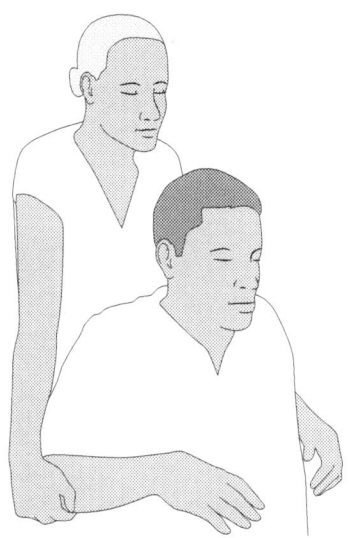

strong likelihood that muscles such as upper trapezius, levator scapulae or rhomboid minor are contributing to the client's problem. They or their surrounding fascia or both may be shortened.

However, if there is little or *no difference* in pain/stiffness or discomfort, and *no increase* in cervical ROM, this suggests that the cervical vertebrae, their discs or their ligaments are contributing to the problem. The rationale for this conclusion is that by reducing tension in the muscles spanning the shoulder-neck region, you would expect there to be a reduction in discomfort if it was originating from tension in these tissues. If there is no reduction in symptoms, the symptoms cannot be originating from these soft tissue structures (although it is likely that if there is an underlying joint problem *some* muscular tension will develop, possibly a movement dysfunction also, and therefore the increased muscular tension and/or shortening of soft tissue will contribute in a minor way to the problem).

Another way to consider this is that, if the problem exists in the joint, passively elevating the shoulders will make no difference: the joint still has to move. If anything, passively elevating the shoulders decreases muscular tension and allows the neck to move further. This may increase tension on the problem joint and can heighten the symptom. That is in fact what often happens: a client with a known cervical joint problem will report that the test mildly increases discomfort or makes no difference to the discomfort, whereas a client with muscular tension in the neck reports a decrease in symptoms—as one might expect when muscular 'pull' is taken out of the equation, albeit slightly.

Tip: One way you could decide for yourself whether this is a useful assessment tool is to carry it out on people who you know have underlying bony or ligamentous problems yet are not contraindicated for assessment.

Passive elevation of the shoulders also lessens the tensional pull on scalenes during active rotation of the neck. Try this for yourself: Look over your right shoulder and as you do so, notice how the anterior left side of your neck feels. Next, ask a colleague to passively elevate your shoulders and repeat the movement. With passive shoulder elevation do you notice less tension in your left scalenes on rotation of your head to the right?

TIP 9 MEASURING NECK AND SHOULDER DISTANCE

Another interesting assessment you can perform is to examine the distance between the widest part of a client's head and the widest part of their shoulders. The method by which this is done provides a helpful visual aid that can be used to help explain to clients the importance of maintaining correct neck alignment while they are sleeping.

You will need a large enough floor space for your client to lie down and for you to kneel beside them. Take a large sheet of paper (or several smaller sheets fixed together) and ask your client to lie down on it in the supine position. Help get your client positioned

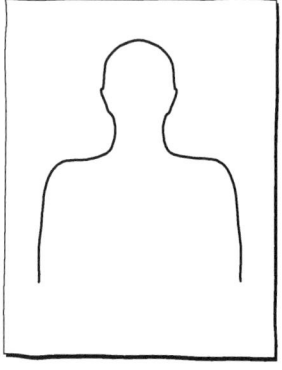

so that their head and shoulders are on the paper. (You do not need their waist or lower part of their body on the paper, just their head and shoulders.) Next, draw around your client, keeping your pen perpendicular to the paper. Draw as close to the client's body as possible. Now ask your client to stand up.

Next, take the image you have drawn and measure the distance between the widest part of the client's head (that is, at the level of the ears) and the widest part of their shoulder. Examine the distance between the head and shoulder. Compare left and right sides. Measure the distance if you want. Are you surprised at how large this distance is? Is it the same on the left and right sides of the client's body?

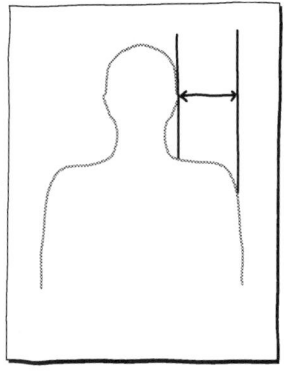

This assessment gives both you and your client a visual understanding of the relationship between their head and neck. This information can be used to show your client how to keep their neck in alignment when sleeping on their side. For more information, please see *Part 3, Tip 6* (pp.256-257).

TIP 10 LOCATING C7 ON YOURSELF

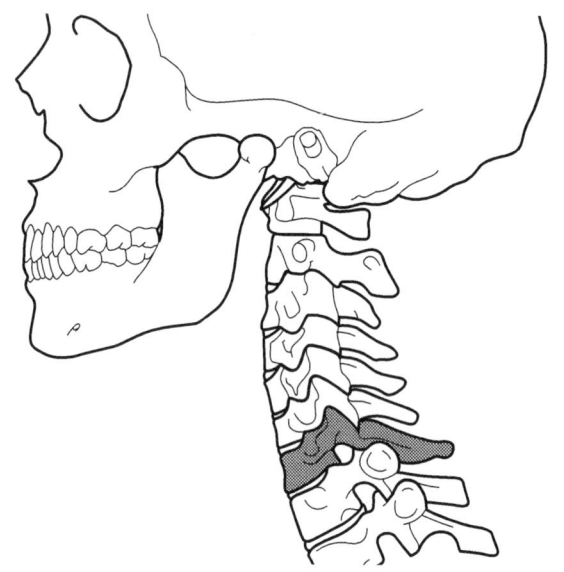

You no doubt remember having to learn anatomy as part of your therapy training, including the names given to groups of different vertebrae (cervical, thoracic, lumbar, sacral, coccygeal), and you may also have learned that these have letters and numbers assigned to them. Cervical vertebrae are assigned the letter 'C' and numbered one to seven, from the top down. The first cervical vertebrae (also known as atlas) is referred to as C1, the second (also known as axis) is referred to as C2. The seventh cervical vertebrae —C7 — is aptly named the *vertebra prominens* because it is the most prominent of the cervical vertebrae and it is a useful bone to be able to locate. Being able to locate this bony prominence gives us a point of reference when assessing and treating clients with neck problems. For example, we can use this point to document whether a tender spot is superior or inferior to C7 and thus be more clear as to the site of a symptom. Should you need to refer a client, being able to describe symptoms in relation to this point may be helpful. For example: "Client reports posterior neck pain on rotation of the head to the right, specific to a point which is level with C7 but approximately 2cm to the right of the C7 spinous process."

Sometimes a client reports a problem in their neck, yet on palpation, you discover the point the client is describing is in the high thoracic region. You know this because you have identified C7 and together you and your client have determined the place the client describes as being inferior to C7. So, being able to locate C7 is useful in order to get a more specific picture of where discomfort may be originating, or where symptoms may manifest.

Try locating C7 on yourself in order to gain confidence in palpating this bony prominence: Place your fingers on the back of your neck, flex your neck and notice that the spinous processes of some vertebrae become prominent. As you move from C7 to C6 to C5 the spinous processes become less distinct and are therefore more difficult to differentiate from one another. In this position, are you able to determine that point on the back of your neck which feels most prominent? Whichever it is, this is likely to be the spinous process of your C7 vertebra.

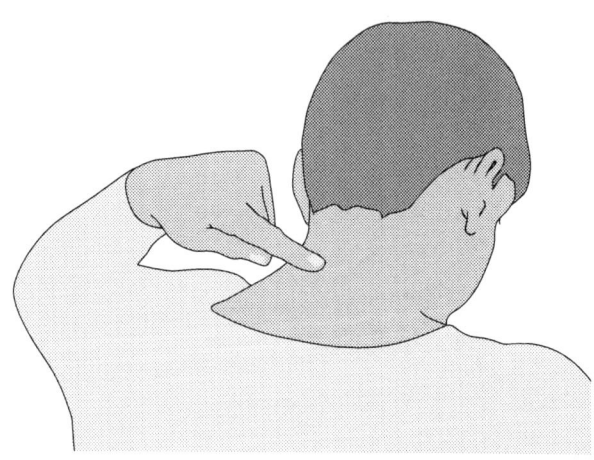

TIP 11 LOCATING C7 ON A CLIENT

This vertebrae may be easily located with the client standing or seated. With your client in the prone position it can sometimes be slightly trickier to identify.

Locating C7 on a standing or seated client
Standing to the side of your client, observe their neck. In many subjects there is a noticeable 'bump' at the base of the neck, made more apparent when they look to the floor, flexing the cervical spine. This bump is C7. When you palpate the back of the neck, the spinous process of C7 is the most prominent. In clients who are very overweight or who have a dowager's hump—with an overgrowth of fatty tissue on the back of the neck—C7 can be harder to see. It seems obvious, but it will also be harder to see in people whose *vertebrae prominens* have shorter, less prominent spinous processes.

Locating C7 on a client in the prone position
When a client rests in the prone position, with their head and face in a neutral position rather than to one side, the neck extends slightly and the spinous processes of the cervical vertebrae approximate

one another. With the neck in slight extension it becomes less easy to distinguish individual vertebrae. Follow these simple steps to help you identify C7 in the prone position.

1. Standing at the head of the couch facing your client's head, place the thumb of your right hand where you think C7 might be (figure 1).
2. Place the thumb of your left hand where you think C6 might be (figure 2).
3. Keeping your thumbs in this position, ask your client to gently lift their head from the couch (figure 3).

Figure 1

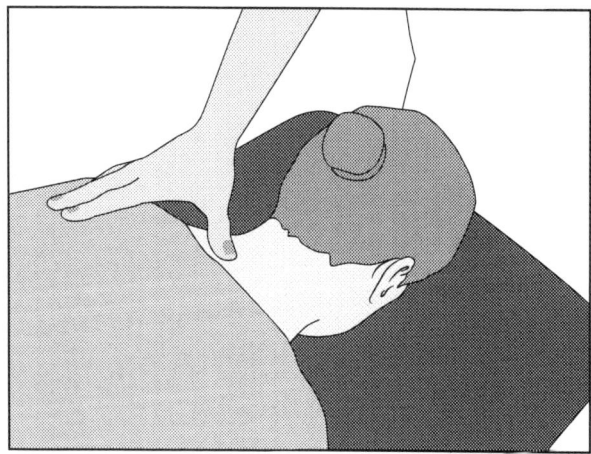

Figure 2

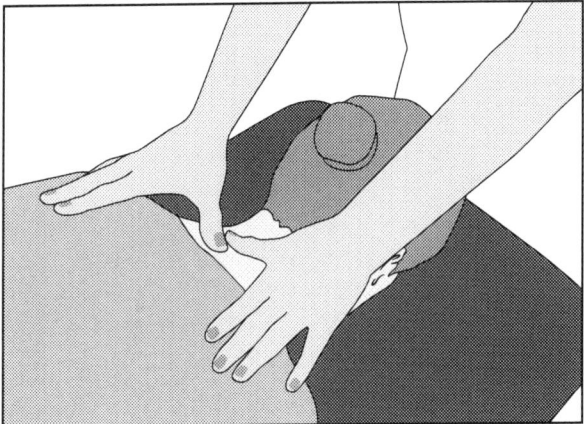

Figure 3

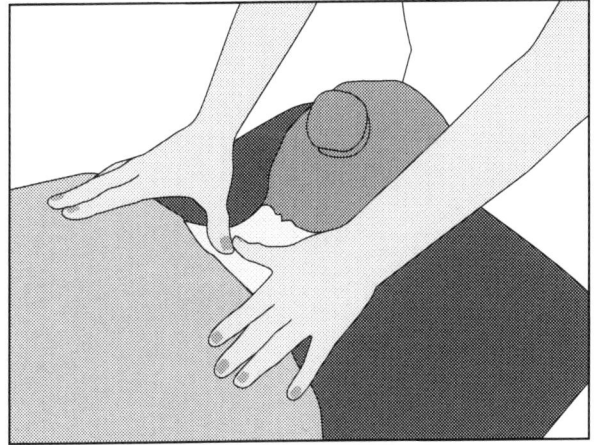

If your right thumb is on C7 you should feel the spinous process of C6 'disappear' beneath your left thumb (figure 4). This is because the spinous processes of the cervical vertebrae approximate one another when the neck is moved into extension, making them more difficult to palpate. C7—at the cervico-

Figure 4

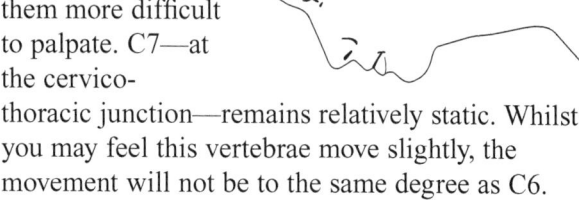

thoracic junction—remains relatively static. Whilst you may feel this vertebrae move slightly, the movement will not be to the same degree as C6.

For a good reference in support of this method of identification, please see Shin S., Yoon D.M., York K.B., 2011. Identification of the correct cervical level by palpation of spinous processes. *Anesth Analog,* May 2011, 112(5):1232-5, Epub 2011 Feb 23.

TIP 12 GETTING GOOD AT LOCATING C7

The shape and prominence of C7 varies considerably between subjects, and you may find that at first you are not sure whether you have correctly identified the vertebrae. There are three ways to confirm you are on C7.

The best way to get good at palpating this bone — or any bony landmark—is simply to practice. Try to find it on a lot of different people. As the saying goes, practice makes perfect.

A second way to improve your skill is to place a mark on C7 with the client sitting, prior to palpation. Using a body crayon, place a dot over this vertebra, which will be more prominent when the client is upright, thus giving you a visual clue when it becomes less prominent as the client assumes the prone position. It's important to note, however, that the dot you mark on the skin with the client seated will not remain in the same position over the vertebrae when the client lies prone, as the skin and soft tissues will move and change as will the vertebrae themselves. Your mark will at least give you a *rough* indication of the lowest point of the cervical spine, and you can use this as a guide.

Thirdly, give this exercise your best attempt by following the steps in *Tip 11* (pp.58-60) and then, using the same client, deliberately place your thumbs in the *wrong* positions: place your right thumb over T1 (instead of C7) and your left thumb over C7 (instead of C6). Ask your subject to once again lift their head off the couch. Change back to the correct positions described in Tip 11—that is, with your right thumb on C7 and your left on C6. Ask your client to lift their head. Compare the difference you feel beneath your thumbs in the 'right' and 'wrong' positions. By making comparisons between how different areas of the neck feel when you palpate C6 and C7 you can eventually decide which is the most *likely* location of C7. The most likely location when palpating in the prone position is when C6 'disappears' beneath your thumb.

TIP 13 IDENTIFYING SCALENES ON YOURSELF

Scalenes are an interesting group of neck muscles because they may be responsible for referring pain to other parts of the body such as the medial border of the scapula (in the location of the rhomboids), the shoulder and the upper limb. Nerves and blood vessels pass down to the upper limb by coursing through a small area which is bordered by the clavicle, ribs, pectoralis minor and scalene muscles.

Compression of the blood vessels or nerves in this area of the neck leads to a range of upper limb symptoms collectively known as *thoracic outlet syndrome*. There is controversy surrounding whether tension in scalenes may contribute to thoracic outlet syndrome. Some therapists find that by

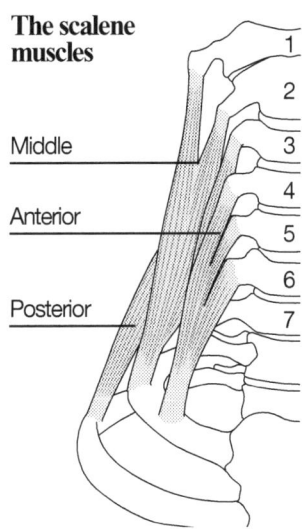

The scalene muscles

Middle

Anterior

Posterior

1
2
3
4
5
6
7

decreasing tension in these muscles—through stretching, massage, trigger point work or repositioning of the head and neck through exercise, for example—symptoms of thoracic outlet syndrome are alleviated in some subjects. Attaching to the first and second ribs, scalenes are also important muscles of respiration. Being able to identify and to palpate them is therefore useful in assessing for muscular tension.

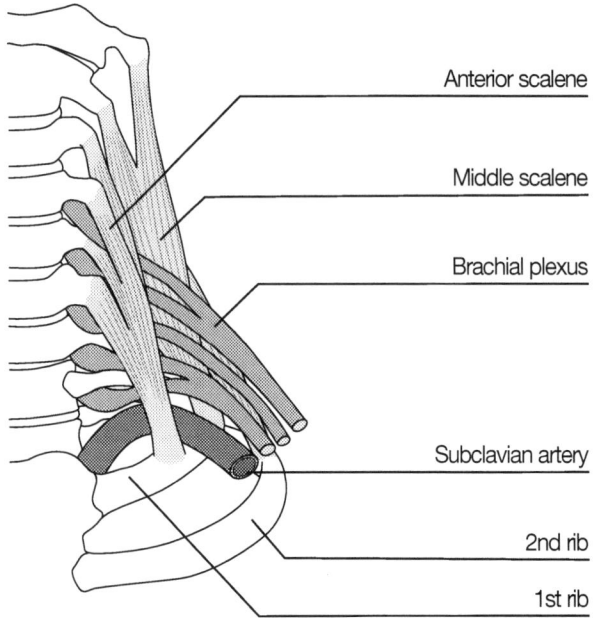

Anterior scalene

Middle scalene

Brachial plexus

Subclavian artery

2nd rib

1st rib

Some people feel anxious about having their neck palpated, especially the anterior aspect. To gain confidence with assessing this sensitive area, follow these steps and practice identifying your own scalenes.

Step 1 Facing a mirror, first identify the two muscles which are *not* scalenes. Draw your mouth downward and locate the flat sheet of the platysma muscle that resembles a turtle's neck. Note that the tendons of this muscle are at the lateral ends of your clavicles.

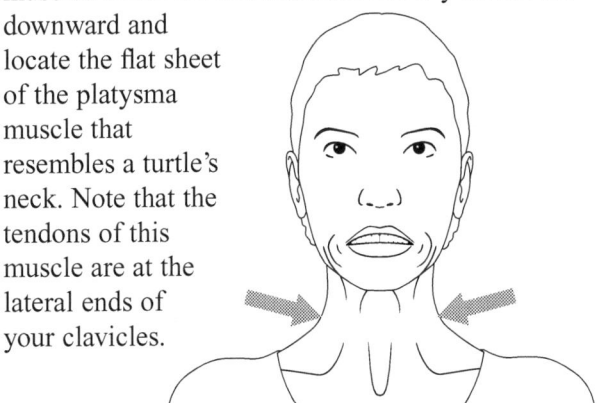

Step 2 Relax your mouth and locate sternocleidomastoid. This muscle rotates the head and neck to the opposite side: the right sternocleidomastoid rotates the head and neck to the left; the left sternocleidomastoid rotates the head and neck to the right. Practice rotating your head one way and then the other until you are sure you have identified this muscle.

Tip: When you gently pinch the muscle at its base where it originates on the sternum and clavicle, you will feel it contract. For example, rotate your head to the left and note that you can feel your right muscle contract.

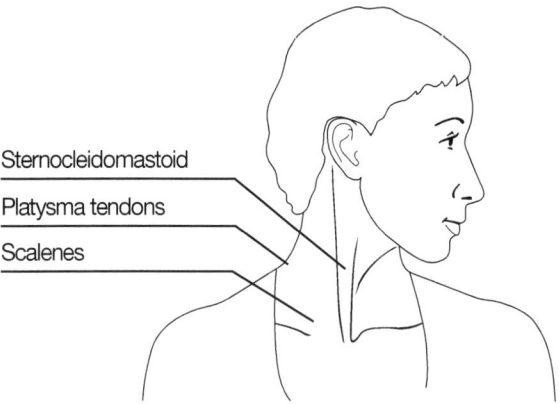

Sternocleidomastoid

Platysma tendons

Scalenes

Step 3 Locate the *position* of scalenes. These are located between the tendons of platysma and the sternocleidomastoid muscle. That is, your right scalene muscles are located between the right platysma tendon and your right sternocleido-mastoid muscle; your left scalene muscles are located between the left platysma tendon and your left sternocleidomastoid muscle.

Step 4 Now that you know the *region* in which to look and palpate for scalenes, let's identify them for sure. Face the mirror and place your right fist against your forehead. Gently push your head into your fist and notice that your scalenes (on both sides) become prominent as they contract. You will see them above your clavicles and just lateral to the sternocleidomastoid on each side, but not as lateral as the tendon of platysma, the 'turtle' neck muscle.

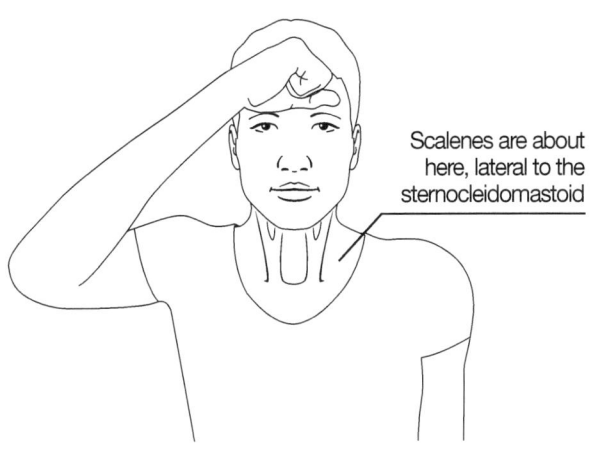

Scalenes are about here, lateral to the sternocleidomastoid

Question: How can I check I have identified my scalene muscles correctly?

The answer is to palpate them while they contract. This is where it is useful to revise some muscle functions. Both scalenes and the sternocleidomastoid bring about neck flexion and so both contract when you press your forehead into your fist as described. However, the right scalenes do *not* contract when you turn your head to the left (whereas the right sternocleidomastoid does) and the left scalenes do *not* contract when you turn your head to the left (whereas the left sternocleidomastoid does). We can use this information to differentiate between scalenes and the sternocleidomastoid.

Differentiating between scalenes and sternocleidomastoid
Step 1 Locate both the right sternocleidomastoid and the right scalenes by observing for and palpating these as they contract on resisted neck flexion. You will see the muscles 'appear' when you press your head into your fist, and you can palpate and 'feel' the increase in tone, demonstrating that both muscles have contracted. Next, you need to do something that is a bit tricky.

Step 2 Place your right hand against the right side of your head and resist right rotation while palpating *both* sternocleidomastoid and scalenes. It may work best if you place your left thumb on the sternocleidomastoid and your left forefinger on the scalenes.

You will feel that one of these muscles contracts on right rotation, but the other does not. That is, as you turn your head to the right, you can feel an increase in tone in only one of the muscles. The right scalenes contract on rotation of the head to the right, but the right sternocleidomastoid does not. Unlike the sternocleidomastoid, scalenes rotate the head and neck *to the same side*, whereas the sternocleidomastoid muscles rotate the head and neck *to the opposite side*. If you have correctly identified your right scalene muscles, you will feel them contract on both neck flexion and rotation of the head to the right.

TIP 14 HOW TO OBSERVE SCALENES ON A CLIENT

Scalenes are deep muscles and should not be apparent when you observe a subject at rest, from the front, although you may see them in clients with certain respiratory disorders (remember these are muscles of respiration) where these muscles have become hypertonic due to the extra workload imposed on them. You may see these muscles in subjects with very low body fat. As you might expect, in such people many muscles become more discernible, not just scalenes. However, in a normal, healthy adult, scalenes should not appear prominent. Look closely to see whether one side appears more pronounced than the other. This may indicate an increase in tone on that side. Such an increase in tone may correspond with symptoms on that side of the body.

Secondly, you could locate these muscles on a client in the same way that you located them on yourself. Ask them to face you and to place their own fist against their forehead and gently resist forward flexion. Observe your subject as you instruct them to perform gentle, resisted neck flexion. As when you tried this exercise yourself,

you should see scalenes on either side of the
client's neck, between the tendon of platysma and
the sternocleidomastoid muscle.

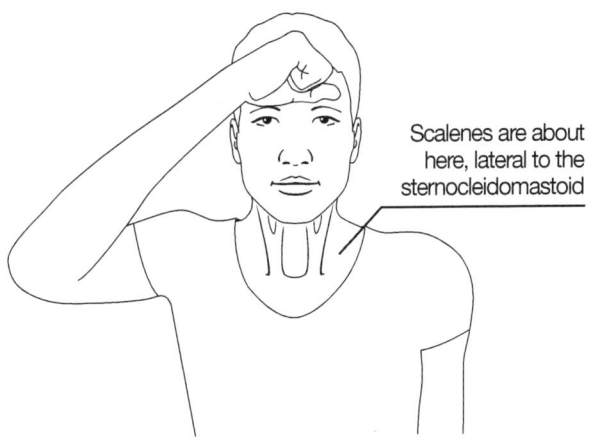

Scalenes are about
here, lateral to the
sternocleidomastoid

Question: What if you wanted to identify scalenes
with your client in the supine position?

Simply ask them to gently lift their head from the
couch and scalenes will be activated and will
become prominent. Lifting the head from the
couch requires flexion of the neck and because the
head is being lifted against gravity, it is not
necessary for the client to press their forehead into
their fist.

TIP 15 HOW TO PALPATE SCALENES ON A CLIENT

There are two ways to do this.

1. Palpating scalenes with your client seated
Stand behind your client and gently palpate the anterior of their neck using light, fingertip touch.

Tip: Use only one hand. Rest your other hand gently on the client's shoulder. The reason for this

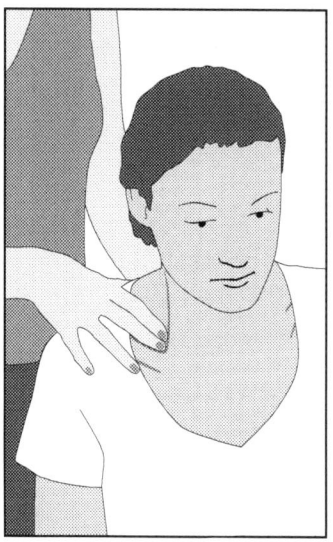

is that it can be unnerving to have someone stand behind you with both hands on your neck, albeit for the purposes of assessment and within a professional capacity. Having both hands around the neck, even with light fingertip touch, could make some clients anxious.

Locate your subject's clavicle and keep your fingers on or superior to this bone.

Ask your client to place one of their fists gently on their forehead and to gently press their forehead into their fist. As you know, both scalenes and the sternocleidomastoid will contract when they do this. Palpate along the clavicle, superior to this bone, feeling for the contraction in scalenes.

From practicing on yourself as described in *Tip 13* (pp.65-69), you now know that only scalenes contract ipsilaterally on rotation. That is, the right scalene contracts on rotation of the head to the right (whereas the sternocleidomastoid does not) and the left scalenes contract on rotation of the head to the left (whereas the left sternocleidomastoid does not). By asking your client to turn their head to the right, for example, you should now be able to identify their right scalene muscles: you should know that they can be palpated superior to the clavicle, close to the bone, in between the sternocleidomastoid muscle and the tendon of platysma.

2. Palpating scalenes with your client supine
It is sometimes easier to palpate scalenes with a
subject supine than it is with them seated.
Standing at the head of the couch, using one hand
only, once again palpate your subject's neck
superior to the clavicle, between the
sternocleidomastoid and the platysma tendon. Ask
your client to lift their head off the couch. Once
again, the scalenes will contract and you should be
able to identify them as an increase in tone
beneath your fingertips.

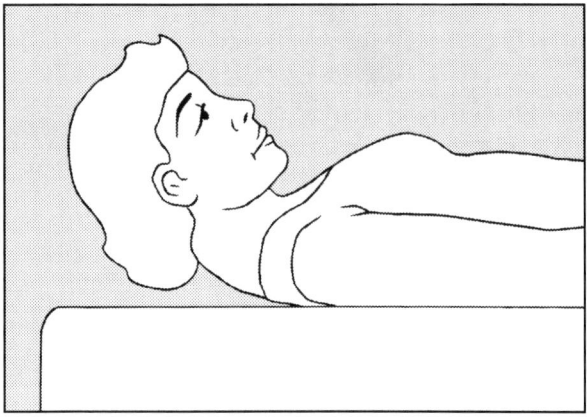

For more information about these fascinating
muscles and tips on how to treat trigger points in
them, turn to *Part 2, Tip 18: Treating Scalenes*
(pp.208-210).

TIP 16 THE TONGUE TEST

In his book *Do-It-Yourself Shiatsu*, Wataru Ohashi says that if you ask a client to stick out their tongue you can determine which side of their neck is 'tight' by the direction the tongue is pointing. A tongue pointing to the right indicates tension in the right side of the neck; a tongue pointing to the left indicates tension in the left side of the neck. Ohashi explains that this is due to muscles pulling on the tongue. What do you think? Are you tempted to try this form of assessment? Although Ohashi doesn't state which muscles are responsible for observed tongue deviation, we know that omohyoid is a strange little strap-like muscle connecting the superior angle of the scapula with the hyoid bone and, as you may remember, the hyoid bone is the bone at the front of the throat anchoring the tongue. As you will learn from *Tip 17*, the shoulder is related to the neck, so it would be interesting to observe whether there is any tongue deviation in clients with shoulder problems. Are you brave enough to include this as a form of assessment!

Ohashi, W., 1977. *Do-It-Yourself Shiatsu*. London: Unwin Paperbacks.

TIP 17 APPRECIATING THE NECK/UPPER LIMB RELATIONSHIP

Place the fingers of your right hand on the back of your neck, in the centre, along the spinous processes of your cervical vertebrae. Now abduct your left arm. Notice that you can feel subtle movement beneath your fingers. Swap hands, this time palpating your neck with the fingers of your left hand while also abducting your right arm. You are likely feeling an increase in tone in trapezius (where it inserts to a soft tissue structure called the ligamentum nuchae running down the spinous processes of the cervical spine), which you may remember spans the posterior of the neck and attaches to the spine of the scapula and which contracts to help bring about movement of the scapula.

So why is this important? The neck and shoulder are connected via a huge array of soft tissues. Whilst the neck is the focus of this book, it's well known that we cannot treat parts of the body in isolation. (Many would argue that we cannot treat *the body* in isolation—the mind must be addressed also.) When a client comes for treatment of a neck problem, assessment of the shoulder is useful—

many would argue essential. Existing or previous
shoulder problems may contribute to a current
neck problem and both of these parts of the body
will need to be addressed if there is to be a
successful resolution.

Therefore, whilst there are time constraints on how
long you can assess and treat a client, it's worth
considering a shoulder assessment if the neck
problem you are treating remains unresolved. In
such cases it is useful to enquire and to reflect on
how your client is using their upper limbs, because
it is impossible to compartmentalize the body in
real life, as you know. Levator scapulae is a
muscle which, when you learn more about it in the
next tip, helps make this point clearer.

TIP 18 WHAT ARE 'KNOTS' IN THE NECK REGION?

If you are used to providing massage for your clients you are likely to have felt some areas of the neck and shoulder to be bumpy or knotty. Experienced therapists know that when 'trigger points' are pressed, they elicit a kind of 'grateful pain'. It may be that you have come across a trigger spot, a small, localized area of tension that when pressed produces this kind of pain. It is important to remember that not all areas of palpable tension are trigger points.

First, they could be normal bony anatomy. Look at a model skeleton and observe how the ribs protrude posteriorly. Though not as likely in the cervical region, it is possible that an area of tension you can feel is in fact a rib. Although rare, a small percentage of the population have a cervical rib that is palpable anteriorly.

Secondly, the area of tension could be normal muscular anatomy. Consider levator scapulae. This muscle originates on the transverse processes of the upper cervical vertebrae and inserts on the superior angle of the scapulae. Notice how it twists back on itself. Could the 'knots' you sometimes feel in this region actually be normal muscular anatomy rather than tense tissues?

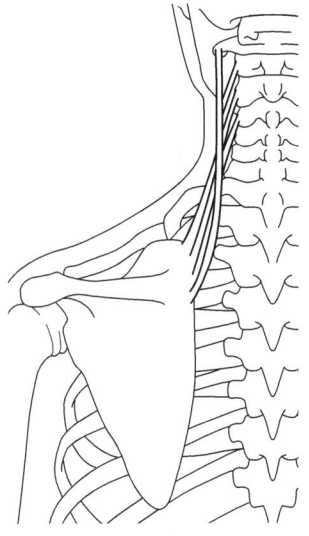

If you suspect levator scapulae *does* contain trigger spots, and that it is not just normal muscular anatomy you can feel, reading *Part 2: Neck Treatment Tips & Tricks* will be helpful as this provides tips on how you can position your client in various ways to gain better access to this muscle.

Thirdly, there are other explanations for palpable lumps, such as lipomas, tumors or scar tissue, for example. The purpose of this book is not to teach diagnostics, and if you have any doubt as to whether the lump you have found is a trigger point or normal musculoskeletal anatomy, you should refer your client to their doctor.

TIP 19 THE IMPORTANCE OF SUBOCCIPITALS

Attaching to either of the first two cervical vertebrae, the four small muscles at the base of the skull that are collectively known as suboccipitals are responsible for rocking and tilting the head. Feel the flicker of your own suboccipitals by placing your fingertips gently beneath the occiput. Now roll your eyes in a circle. Can you feel your suboccipitals flickering? One of these muscles is known as rectus capitis posterior minor and is particularly curious because it has a high proportion of muscle spindles. Muscles with a high proportion of spindles are involved in proprioception. So atrophy of this muscle in clients following injury (such as whiplash) may be significant and may contribute to a reduced sense of balance.

Rectus capitis posterior minor is also important because it is connected to the dura mater of the brain via a layer of fascia. Tension and the development of trigger points in suboccipitals may be one explanation for tension headaches, as increased tension is transmitted to the dura via this fascial connection.

Further, as injury or atrophy of suboccipitals could affect balance, these muscles may contribute to hamstring tension. For a discussion of this point see McPartland *et al* (1997) and Moseley (2004).

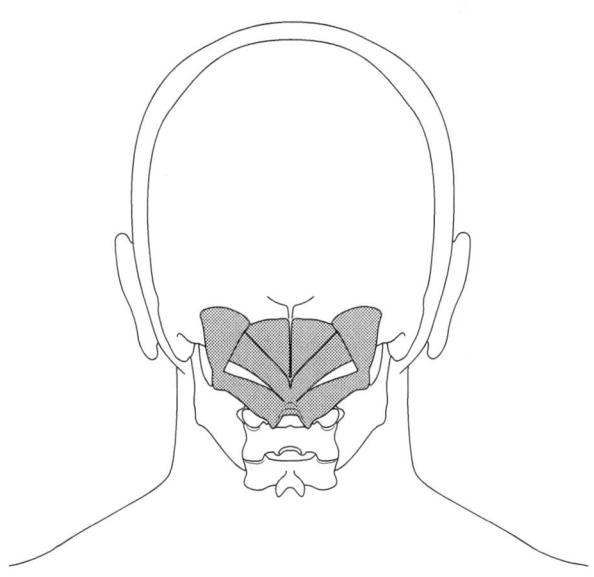

For further information, see McPartland, J.M., Brodeur, R.R. and Hallgren, R.C., 1997. Chronic neck pain, standing balance, and suboccipital muscle atrophy – a pilot study. *Journal of Manipulative and Physiological Therapeutics, 20(1): 24-9.* Also see Moseley, G.L., 2004. Impaired trunk muscle function in patients with sub-acute neck pain: etiologic in the subsequent development of low-back pain. *Manual Therapy, 9:157-163.*

TIP 20 PALPATING SUBOCCIPITALS

It is difficult effectively to palpate these muscles as they lie deep to trapezius and the thick fascia of the posterior of the neck. One way to palpate the posterior neck is with the client prone. However, if they try to turn their head, they need to lift it, extending the neck; muscles of the posterior neck become tense, thereby making palpation difficult. An alternative is to position your client supine. Practice palpating the posterior neck in these positions and see which works best for you.

a) Client prone, you at the head of the couch

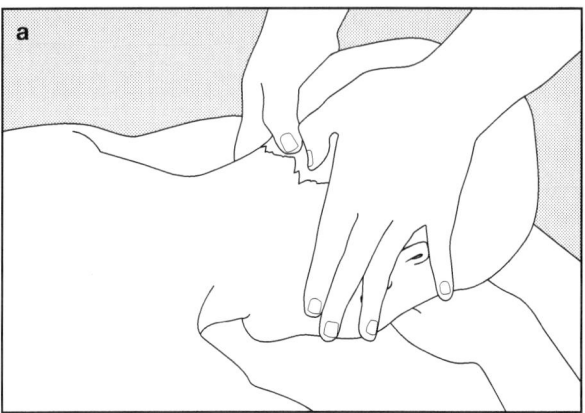

b) Client supine, you standing at the head of the couch with your hands either side of the client's neck

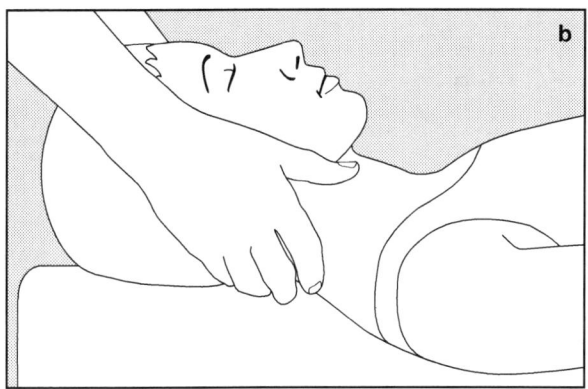

c) Client supine, you facing your client with your hands either side of their neck

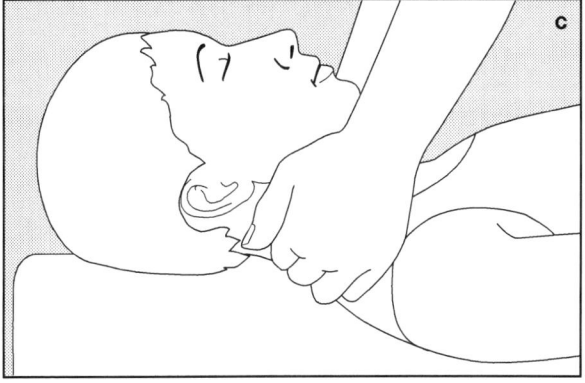

d) Client supine, you standing at the head of the couch, cupping the base of the skull

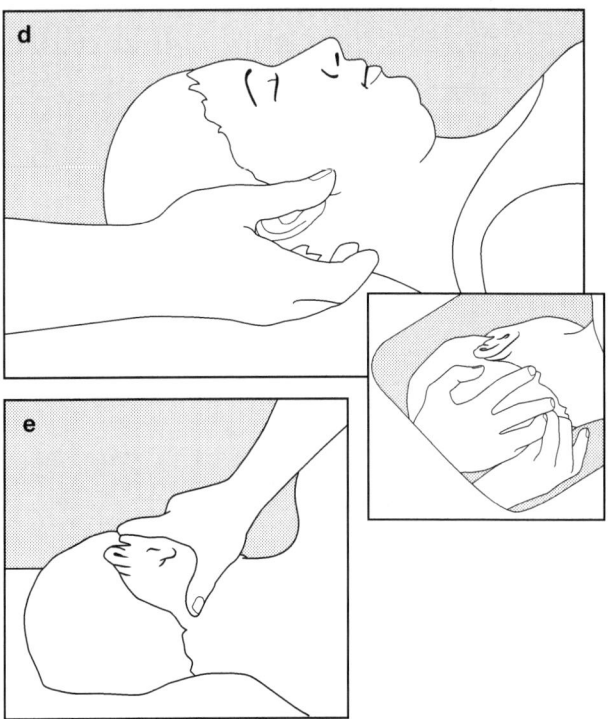

e) Client side lying, you standing behind them

TIP 21 CLIENT PERCEPTIONS OF PAIN

In *Tip 7: Documenting Discomfort* (pp.44-46),
you read about the importance of documenting the
terminology used by clients to report their
symptoms. It is also important to consider how a
neck problem impacts on the activities of daily life
for a person—how it affects their work, family life
and participation in hobbies. Based on the
Oswestry Low Back Pain Disability Questionnaire
(Fairbanks *et al*), The Neck Disability Index
(NDI) is a questionnaire designed to measure
self-perceived disability resulting from neck pain.
A similar questionnaire was designed by the
team at Northwick Park Hospital in England and
is called the Northwick Park Neck Pain
Questionnaire (NPQ). Both of these questionnaires
comprise a series of questions which cover pain
intensity, personal care (washing, dressing, etc),
lifting, reading, headaches, concentration, work,
driving, sleeping and recreation.

Fairbanks, J.C., Couper, J., Davies, J.B., O'Brien, J.P., 1980. The
Oswestry Low Back Pain Disability Questionnaire. *Physiotherapy*, 1980;
66:271-273

Leak, A.M., Cooper, J., Dyer, S., Williams, K.A., Turner-Stokes, L., Frank,
A.O.,1994. The Northwick Park neck pain questionnaire, devised to
measure neck pain and disability. *Br. J. Rheumatol.*, 1994; 33:469–474.

The purpose of such questionnaires is to help identify the level of disability that the neck problem represents to a client. The results serve as a baseline marker and enable practitioners to identify whether their interventions are reducing the overall level of disability that the client perceives themselves to have.

Examining the validity of these questionnaires for use with patients suffering from Whiplash Associated Disorders (WAD), researchers Hoving et al (2003) noted that the questionnaires omitted emotional and social items judged to be important to patients. Nevertheless, you could use the subheadings from the questionnaires as a prompt when assessing your own clients to determine how their neck condition impacts on their daily life. A sample prompt sheet has been provided for you on the next page.

Hoving, J.L., O'Leary, E.F., Niere, K.R., Green, S., Buchbinder, R., 2003. Validity of the neck disability index, Northwick Park neck pain questionnaire, and problem elicitation technique for measuring disability associated with whiplash-associated disorders. *Pain*, 102(3): 273-281

Activity	Comments
Personal care	
Lifting	
Reading	
Headaches	
Concentration	
Work	
Driving	
Sleeping	
Recreation	

TIP 22 NECK DISABILITY INDEX

Vernon and Mior (1991) developed a questionnaire called The Neck Disability Index. They considered how a neck problem affects people in terms of what most people do on a daily basis, during an average day. To assess this, they devised a series of questions which they grouped into ten sections:

Section 1: Pain Intensity
Section 2: Personal Care (Washing, Dressing, etc.)
Section 3: Lifting
Section 4: Reading
Section 5: Headaches
Section 6: Concentration
Section 7: Work
Section 8: Driving
Section 9: Sleeping
Section 10: Recreation

By asking people to answer the questions within each section of the questionnaire clinicians get a better idea of how a person's neck problem affects their ability to cope with the activities of daily life. The answers to these questions are assigned numerical values which mean they can be tallied and used to come up with an overall score. This makes it possible to use the neck disability index to help measure change over time, to determine whether a particular intervention has been useful.

I'm not a doctor or neck specialist so is it still worth using the questionnaire?

One way you to utilize this questionnaire is to help clients identify where they *don't* have a problem, which aspects of their daily life are *not* affected by their neck pain. Helping clients to identify pain-free times of their day and the activities they can perform pain-free can be very empowering. Another way you could use it is to prompt your own thinking and to trigger lines of enquiry. For example, if 'section 4: reading' is scored highly you could explore whether it makes a difference in which position your client reads – sitting on a high backed chair or sitting up in bed, for example – or could ask whether it makes a difference how heavy the book is, or whether they hold it on their lap or on a book rest. A client who reports pain in their neck from reading journal articles while sitting at a desk may not get the same pain when they hold the lightweight journal in front of them. The kind of information that can be generated by using this questionaire is invaluable in helping clients to find ways to manage their pain.

If you want to try this questionnaire you could practice by using it with a family member or friend whom you know has had neck problems. Ask them to read the simple instructions and then complete the questionnaire. You will need to read the instructions at the end of the questionnaire that tell you how to create a 'score' (see pp.96-97).

Once you have read the instructions and understand how to use the Neck Disability Index you could use the chart on the opposite page to record the scores for five people you know who have a neck problem. Compare the numerical results. Those with a higher percentage score are classed as having a higher level of neck-related disability. Do you agree with this? Would you say that your subjects who rated more highly have a higher level of disability? Another useful comparison might be to examine five people you know have had a common neck-related disorder such as whiplash or a trapped nerve.

Practising With the Neck Disability Index Score

Subject	Neck Disability Index Score	Comments
Subject 1		
Subject 2		
Subject 3		
Subject 4		
Subject 5		

Vernon, H., and Mior, S., 1991. The Neck Disability Index: A study of reliability and validity. *Journal of Manipulative and Physiological Therapeutics*, 14, 409-415

Neck Disability Index

Information for clients: This questionnaire has been designed to help me understand how your neck pain has affected your ability to manage in everyday life. Please answer every section and in each section mark ONE box that applies to you. If you consider that two or more statements in any one section relate to you, please mark the box that most closely describes your problem.

Section 1: Pain Intensity
❏ I have no pain at the moment
❏ The pain is very mild at the moment
❏ The pain is moderate at the moment
❏ The pain is fairly severe at the moment
❏ The pain is very severe at the moment
❏ The pain is the worst imaginable at the moment

Section 2: Personal Care (Washing, Dressing, etc.)
❏ I can look after myself normally without causing extra pain
❏ I can look after myself normally but it causes extra pain
❏ It is painful to look after myself and I am slow and careful
❏ I need some help but can manage most of my personal care
❏ I need help every day in most aspects of self care
❏ I do not get dressed, I wash with difficulty and stay in bed

Section 3: Lifting

❑ I can lift heavy weights without extra pain
❑ I can lift heavy weights but it gives extra pain
❑ Pain prevents me lifting heavy weights off the floor, but I can manage if they are conveniently placed, for example on a table
❑ Pain prevents me from lifting heavy weights but I can manage light to medium weights if they are conveniently positioned
❑ I can only lift very light weights
❑ I cannot lift or carry anything

Section 4: Reading

❑ I can read as much as I want to with no pain in my neck
❑ I can read as much as I want to with slight pain in my neck
❑ I can read as much as I want to with moderate pain in my neck
❑ I can't read as much as I want to because of moderate pain in my neck
❑ I can hardly read at all because of severe pain in my neck
❑ I cannot read at all

Section 5: Headaches

❑ I have no headaches at all
❑ I have slight headaches, which come infrequently
❑ I have moderate headaches, which come infrequently
❑ I have moderate headaches, which come frequently

❏ I have severe headaches, which come frequently
❏ I have headaches almost all the time

Section 6: Concentration
❏ I can concentrate fully when I want to with no difficulty
❏ I can concentrate fully when I want to with slight difficulty
❏ I have a fair degree of difficulty in concentrating when I want to
❏ I have a lot of difficulty in concentrating when I want to
❏ I have a great deal of difficulty in concentrating when I want to
❏ I cannot concentrate at all

Section 7: Work
❏ I can do as much work as I want to
❏ I can only do my usual work, but no more
❏ I can do most of my usual work, but no more
❏ I cannot do my usual work
❏ I can hardly do any work at all
❏ I can't do any work at all

Section 8: Driving
❏ I can drive my car without any neck pain
❏ I can drive my car as long as I want to with slight pain in my neck
❏ I can drive my car as long as I want to with moderate pain in my neck

❑ I can't drive my car as long as I want to because of moderate pain in my neck

❑ I can hardly drive at all because of severe pain in my neck

❑ I can't drive my car at all

Section 9: Sleeping

❑ I have no trouble sleeping

❑ My sleep is slightly disturbed (less than 1 hr sleepless)

❑ My sleep is mildly disturbed (1-2 hrs sleepless)

❑ My sleep is moderately disturbed (2-3 hrs sleepless)

❑ My sleep is greatly disturbed (3-5 hrs sleepless)

❑ My sleep is completely disturbed (5-7 hrs sleepless)

Section 10: Recreation

❑ I am able to engage in all my recreation activities with no neck pain at all

❑ I am able to engage in all my recreation activities, with some pain in my neck

❑ I am able to engage in most, but not all of my usual recreation activities because of pain in my neck

❑ I am able to engage in a few of my usual recreation activities because of pain in my neck

❑ I can hardly do any recreation activities because of pain in my neck

❑ I can't do any recreation activities at all

How to score the Neck Disability Index

Each of the 10 sections is scored separately (0 to 5 points each) and then added up (max. total = 50). Note that whilst there are six questions within each section, the first question scores zero. If the first statement is ticked, the section score = 0, if the last statement is ticked, it = 5.

EXAMPLE:
Section 3: Lifting
❏ I can lift heavy weights without extra pain (0)
❏ I can lift heavy weights but it gives extra pain (1)
❏ Pain prevents me lifting heavy weights off the floor, but I can manage if they are conveniently placed, for example on a table (2)
❏ Pain prevents me from lifting heavy weights but I can manage light to medium weights if they are conveniently positioned (3)
❏ I can only lift very light weights (4)
❏ I cannot lift or carry anything (5)

If all 10 sections are completed, double the client's score to get a percentage figure.

Example 1: if you add up the scores and this equals 30, 30 x 2 = 60. So their percentage disability is 60%;

Example 2: if their total score is 12, 12 x 2 = 24. So their percentage disability is 24%.

The higher the percentage the more the neck problem is affecting the client in their daily life.

What if I have a client who cannot complete all of the sections, can I still use the questionnaire?
Yes. If you were treating a client who cannot drive, for example, they will not be able to complete section 8.

To calculate the score when a section cannot be completed or has been omitted, divide the patient's total score by the number of sections completed times 5.

$$\frac{\text{PATIENT'S SCORE}}{\text{\# OF SECTIONS COMPLETED} \times 5} \times 100 = \quad \text{\% DISABILITY}$$

Example 1
If 9 of 10 sections are completed, and the score is 30:

$$\frac{30}{9 \times 5} \times 100 = 66.66\% \text{ disability}$$

$$\frac{30}{45} \times 100 = 66.66\%$$

Example 2
If 9 out of 10 sections are completed and the score is 22:

$$\frac{22}{9 \times 5} \times 100 = 48\% \text{ disability}$$

TIP 23 POSTURAL ASSESSMENT REMINDER

Here is a reminder about some of the things you may choose to look for in a postural assessment of the head and neck.

Ear level	Head and neck tilt
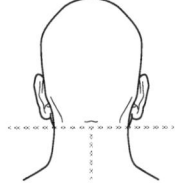	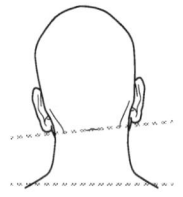
Uneven ear level could mean that the client's head and neck are laterally flexed to one side, or simply that they have one ear positioned higher than the other. Where the latter is the case, clients often know this because they report finding it difficult to get glasses to sit properly.	Clients observed to have lateral neck flexion when resting are likely to have shortened muscles on the side to which they are flexed, notably levator scapulae, scalenes, sternocleidomastoid, and the upper fibers of trapezius on that side of the body.

For full descriptions of what to look for in a postural assessment of the neck region see *Postural Assessment* by Jane Johnson, 2012.

Johnson, J, *Postural Assessment,* 2012. Champaign, IL: Human Kinetics

Head and neck rotation	Cervical spine alignment
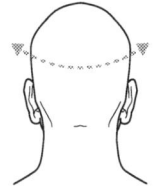	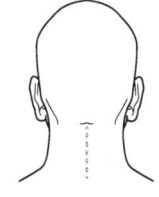
Can you see more of one side of your client's face than the other? More of their jaw or eyelashes on one side? A client who appears to be rotated to the right when relaxed could have shortened scalenes and levator scapulae on that side, and an increase in tone in the sternocleidomastoid on the left side of their neck.	It is also worth checking to see whether the cervical spine itself appears to be in alignment. Does it appear vertical? Are there any marks or swelling present? How do the paraspinal muscles running up the back of the neck appear—are they very prominent? Are muscles on both sides even in tone?

Notice from these illustrations how small lateral deviations in the neck significantly alter the angle between the upper cervical vertebrae and the skull. Where there is a decrease in angle, (a), tissues will be shortened; where there is an increase in angle, (b), they will be lengthened. These findings may help explain a client's symptoms and will help inform your treatment.

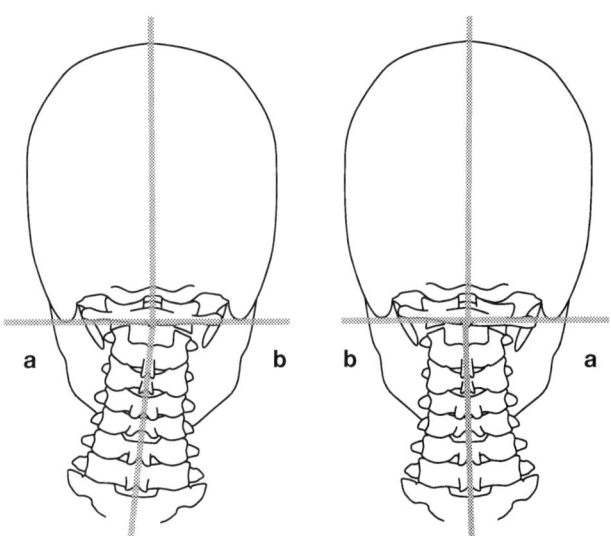

a   b   b   a

The forward head posture describes a type of posture in which the head is carried in advance of the body. The head weighs about 5kg (11 lbs) and should rest directly over the thorax so that the weight of the head is supported by the slightly lordotic curve of the cervical vertebrae. However, as your head moves forward, muscles on the posterior of your neck (levator scapulae, for example) have to work extremely hard. This is fine for everyday movements of the head and neck, into and out of flexion and extension, but is not good when the head remains in the forward position. When the head rests in the forward position, posterior cervical muscles are required to maintain this position and begin to fatigue, and tissues become lengthened and stressed. This is one of the reasons people with this type of posture experience pain in the neck and shoulders.

As muscles of the posterior of the neck lengthen and fatigue they weaken. Anterior neck muscles may become shortened and weak, as they too are held in a less than optimal position. The result is altered head and neck biomechanics and this has a knock-on effect to other parts of the body. Other parts of the spine are then strained as they struggle to counterbalance a heavy head that is being held too far forward and is not being supported through the midline of the body. It is for this reason that many therapists argue that treatments to the thorax and lumbar spine have short-lived effects if the neck and head position are not also addressed in people with thoracic and lumbar problems. We do not know whether the maintenance of a forward head posture *causes* low back pain, but it seems reasonable to assume that such a posture could certainly *aggravate* dysfunction in the lumbar region.

Head position	Cervicothoracic junction
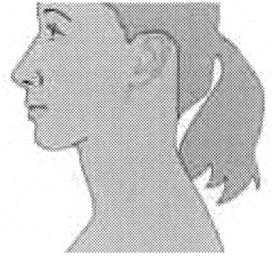	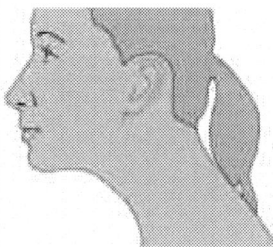

Does the head appear to sit over the thorax or is it pushed forward? Such a posture causes levator scapulae to become hypertonic as it struggles to maintain and move the head in a less than optimal manner, often having to work isometrically. In such a posture the suboccipitals are also stressed as they work to tilt the head backwards so that the eyes are facing forwards, and often clients with such a posture experience tenderness when the suboccipitals are palpated and massaged.	Look at the position of C7. Does there appear to be an abnormal overgrowth of fatty tissue here? This is frequently observed in people with forward head postures where there is a raised portion of tissue over the C7/T1 junction.

Question: What causes this deposit of fatty tissue? It is not clear whether this is hormonal (it is frequently seen in women) or the result of an altered posture and less efficient neck-thorax biomechanics. |

Head position	**Clavicles**
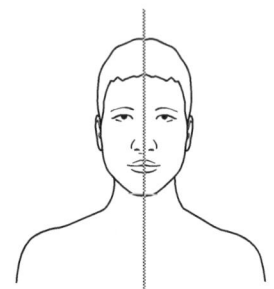	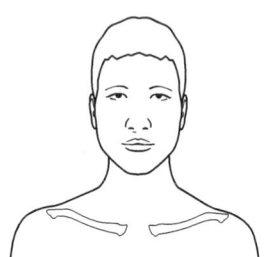
Does the head sit comfortably over the thorax? Is the nose aligned over the manubrium? Is any rotation or lateral tilt that was observed posteriorly also evident in an anterior observation?	Are the clavicles even in both height and orientation? How sharp is the angle they form from the sternoclavicular joint? The smaller the angle the higher the shoulder on that side. Do they have smooth contours?

Muscle tone	Shoulder level
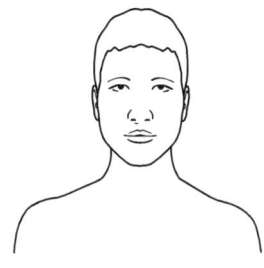	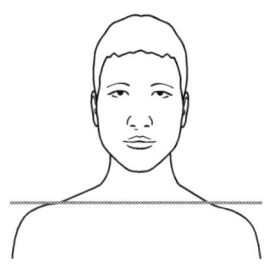
Can you see the scalene muscles? Or see the sternocleidomastoid? Is there an increase in tone in muscles on one side of the neck compared to the other? Prominence in the appearance of these muscles can indicate a forward head posture or chronic respiratory condition.	It is impossible to separate the neck from the shoulder region so any observation of the neck should also take into account the position of the shoulders both anteriorly, posteriorly and when the client is viewed from the side.

TIP 24 FUNCTIONAL STRENGTH TESTING

Cervical strength is usually tested by the examiner holding the client's head still while the client attempts to move their head through each of the cervical ranges, one at a time. The examiner notes the strength the client exerts, whether this appears to fall within a normal range for someone of their age, whether there are any obvious weaknesses or differences between left and right sides, and whether such resistance provokes any of the client's symptoms. However, such tests tend to fall within the remit of physiotherapists, osteopaths and sports therapists rather than massage therapists.

One of the simplest and safest methods to assess the strength of neck muscles is to ask a client to perform active neck movements against gravity. The table here shows four different test positions and the muscles that are required to bring about the movement in each position. A client should be able to repeat the movement 6-8 times. Being able to repeat the movement only one or two times indicates weakness in one or more of the muscles associated with this movement.

Position	Movement	Muscles responsible
Supine	Neck flexion	Sternocleidomastoid Scalenes Longus colli Longus capitis
Prone	Neck extension	Splenius capitis Suboccipitals Longissimus Levator scapulae Semispinalis (capitis and cervicis) Upper fibers of trapezius
Side lying	Lateral flexion	Trapezius Levator scapulae Scalenes Sternocleidomastoid Splenius capitis
Supine	Rotation	Sternocleidomastoid Splenius capitis Semispinalis cervicis Suboccipitals Trapezius

Part 2 Neck Treatment
Tips & Tricks

If you have been struggling to achieve the results you want when treating clients with neck problems, or if you simply want some additional treatment ideas, consider using some of the techniques described in this part of the book, the theme of which is *less is more*. Many of the tips you will find here encourage you to relax, to become focused, and to explore the subtle changes that occur in the body as the result of very light touch. When you try a different technique to one you have been using, you tend to work cautiously and are therefore likely to sense gentle, minor movements of the body and in body tissues. Although subtle, these changes can be positive and are often profound. You may discover that by doing *less*, you facilitate an 'allowing' of relaxation and this helps to stimulate the repair process. Adopting a lighter touch, you might achieve greater success with a client than if you try to 'worry' away tension, pain, stiffness or discomfort with an overuse of manual techniques.

Other tips in this section encourage you to consider changing the position in which you treat a client, and some tips provide ideas for treating specific muscles such as suboccipitals, scalenes and sternocleidomastoid.

If you are reading this as a massage therapist, you may be pleased to know that there is evidence to show that massage is effective for the treatment of neck pain. For examples of research papers examining the use of massage for neck pain see Sherman *et al* (2009) and Ezzo *et al* (1976).

Sherman, K.J., Cherkin, D.C., Hawkes, R.J., Miglioretti, D.L., Deyo, R.A., 2009. Randomized trial of therapeutic massage for chronic neck pain. *Clinical Journal of Pain,* 2009, 25:233-238.

Ezzo, J., Haraldsson, B.G., Gross, A.R., Myers, C.D., Morien, A., Goldsmith, et al,1976. Massage for mechanical neck disorders: a systematic review. *Spine* (1976, Philadelphia, PA) 2007, 32:353-362.

TIP 1 LESS IS MORE

Have you ever treated a client with a neck problem which at first seemed to improve but for whom over time, your results began to plateau? Have you ever found yourself repeating the same kind of treatment with a client, hoping that things would improve whilst being secretly frustrated that you weren't making better progress? Perhaps there have been times when you have utilized every technique you know, exhausting your entire armoury of skills, yet the improvements you were hoping for were not forthcoming. It can be tricky to know quite what to do in such situations.

Usually there is *some* progress, and so it is tempting to keep going, to keep providing the same treatment or advice, hoping that there will be a breakthrough sometime soon and that your client will turn up for a session saying, "Hey! After that last treatment I wasn't expecting anything different and yet when I woke up on Sunday I could look over my left shoulder again!" After all, we frequently tell our clients that it can take weeks or even months to resolve a problem, that a neck problem which has built up over many years is not likely to be resolved in a just a few treatment sessions. So with our client's best interests at heart we begin with what we imagine will be a program of treatment, some point in which we will identify a time when the client will no longer need us; a time when they will be able to manage their condition themselves, or their symptoms will resolve entirely. Yet you may have experienced a situation where you at first seemed to make good progress, with the client reporting immediate relief from symptoms, but with successive treatment sessions there was less and less improvement. If this happens towards the end of a successful treatment program, that is good, and one might expect the degree of change to be less with time anyway. There is often a gradual tailing-off of treatment as the client's condition improves and they are naturally weaned off us. But if this slowing down in improvement occurs before a reasonable relief from pain, stiffness or other troubling symptoms, it can be frustrating for you as a therapist. There is always the feeling that we ought to do more, that we *want* to do more. The good news is that, if the treatment you currently provide for a client is proving ineffective, there are many things you could do instead of continuing with the same treatment.

Here are 8 examples:

1. Re-assess your client

You could re-assess your client, right from the beginning, re-evaluating their range and quality of movement, and asking questions to determine whether anything has changed in their work, hobbies or lifestyle that may be relevant to the symptoms they are currently experiencing. The client may be doing something that they do not consider affects their neck, and so has not thought to tell you about it. This could be something quite simple, like deciding to watch an entire series of their favourite TV drama, or to read *War and Peace* cover to cover, or to knit a king size blanket. All of these examples require the maintenance of a static neck posture which for most of us, is not a good thing. Static postures are likely to aggravate some neck problems. Being able to identify an ongoing aggravating factor is very helpful so reassessment is useful. The tips in *Part I* of this book provide over 20 further ideas for how you might assess your client. Could any of these be useful to you?

2. Consult a colleague

With permission from your client, you could enlist a colleague to carry out the re-assessment. Perhaps a colleague will identify something you have missed? They may use a different handhold, or phrase a question in a such a way as to elicit a different reply; they may perform a test with a subtle change, or palpate more firmly (or less firmly). It is always worth asking for a 'second opinion' because a colleague sometimes has a different 'take' on things. Observing how another therapist performs a neck assessment can be a valuable learning experience in itself.

3. Brainstorm

Maintaining the confidentiality of your client, you could brainstorm the problem with other therapists, asking for their advice. Someone might suggest an assessment, treatment or technique you had not considered and which could prove helpful. Perhaps a colleague has even treated a client with a similar condition? In what ways was it similar? In what ways did it differ? What did they do that was helpful?

4. Explore internet forums for information

The value of sharing information about treatments that have proved effective cannot be overestimated. Sometimes this information can be gleaned from colleagues, or you may find it on an internet forum. Whilst you do need to be discerning in which pieces of information to accept, forums are a useful way of sharing information and much can be learned from reading the comments posted by forum users.

5. Consider referral

You could refer your client to a more experienced practitioner, or to a different health professional entirely. It may be that your client has a condition that is not treatable with your particular therapy, or a condition of which you are not aware. Having to refer a client shows you are putting their needs before your own and should be regarded as a strength rather than a weakness.

> *Question*: How long should you wait before referring a client to another practitioner?
>
> This is a difficult question to answer definitively as this depends on the nature and severity of the symptoms as well as on any protocols set out by your governing body or insurance provider. Your answer must depend on what you consider likely to give your client the best treatment outcome.

6. Avoid hands-on treatment entirely

If you feel that you have correctly assessed your client, that there is no need for referral and you do not wish to discuss treatment options with another therapist, another option is for you to do less with the neck, instead of more. At the extreme end of the scale, you could avoid any hands-on treatment entirely. Consider all of the aftercare tips provided in *Part 3* of this book and select those that you feel might be appropriate for your client. Use the information in these tips to provide your client with the means to self-manage their condition while you remain on-hand to offer advice.

7. Reduce your pressure

Sometimes, we risk over-treating. That is, we try to do too much, too soon, perhaps because we are so eager to help. Or, we use too much pressure during a particular treatment session. Sometimes the client enjoys the sensation of deep pressure; sometimes it provides the results we seek; sometimes we feel that by 'working' an area it will improve, especially if at the assessment stage we discover there to be a palpable increase in muscle tone. If you are providing massage, try lightening your touch by half, so that the pressure of your strokes is halved. Then lighten the depth of your touch by half again. If you are a therapist used to using a lot of pressure it can be difficult to change your approach, especially if you have achieved good results in the past with deep tissue massage. Yet sometimes, if we step back, take a breather, and choose to work with *less* effort, our treatment outcomes improve. This may be because by working more slowly, more gently, with far more patience, we become attuned to the nature of the problem. By sitting very still, with a lightness of touch that is only just perceptible, the clients with whom we are working may begin to find the emotional space to help bring about the healing they need.

8. Change your focus

You could consider treating a different part of your client's body altogether. Sometimes, working away from the problem area rather than directly over it, brings about unexpected and positive results. An example of how this might work is provided in *Tip 2*, where you will learn how to facilitate an increase in neck range of movement by treating the shoulder and not the neck.

TIP 2 GENTLE SHOULDER TRACTION TO INCREASE NECK MOBILITY

Let's put this 'less-is-more' approach into practice immediately. A good example of how a less-is-more approach might work is to imagine you are going to treat a client with tension in muscles of their neck. You know that the neck and shoulder cannot really be isolated anatomically, owing to the large number of structures which connect these two parts of the body to each other and also connect them to the face, skull, upper limb, and thorax.

Question: What are some examples of structures which connect the neck and shoulder?

Omohyoid is a strap-like muscle connecting the scapulae to the hyoid bone at the front of the throat; the upper fibers of trapezius connect the scapulae, clavicle, cervical vertebrae and occiput; the brachial plexus is a group of nerves in the armpit originating from the cervical region; the fascia of the deltoid links the fascia of the chest and neck and arm; skin of the shoulder is continuous with skin of the neck, chest and face.

So, by reducing tension in the shoulder you may help to reduce tension in the neck via these interconnected structures. Stretching often alleviates muscular tension but instead of stretching the neck, how about gently stretching some of the tissues connecting the shoulder and the neck, without touching the neck itself at all? This doesn't have to be the *only* treatment you provide—you could also stretch the neck, massage the neck, and use any of the other techniques familiar to you. It is good, however, sometimes to start with something very simple, and experience just how beneficial this can be *before* moving on to more direct techniques.

> *Question:* If the results are positive after this simple stretch, is there a need to do further treatment to the neck?
>
> You may decide that there is no need to do further work, to apply further techniques. Sometimes it is best to let the treatment take effect and to reassess a client the following day or in a few days' time. It can be suprising how effective these non-direct techniques can be.

To perform a simple shoulder-neck stretch, read the question concerning contraindications and if you feel that it is appropriate for your client, follow these steps.

Question: Are there any clients for whom this is specifically contraindicated?

Yes, this would not be appropriate for clients with subluxing or dislocating shoulders, with known hypermobility syndromes or recent trauma to the neck or shoulder.

Step 1 Position your client comfortably in the supine position and stand to one side of the treatment couch. Avoid use of a pillow beneath the head if possible. Gently take hold of the client's arm, keeping it close to their body. In a moment you are going to apply *gentle* traction to the

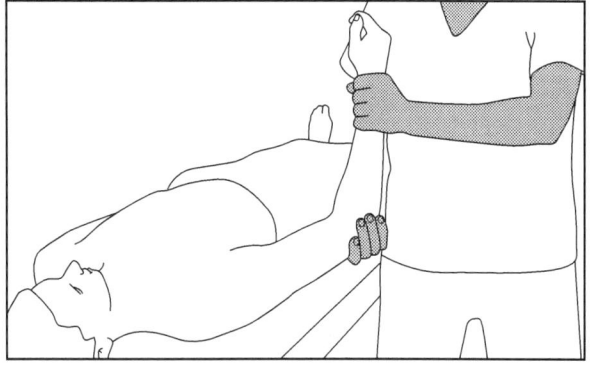

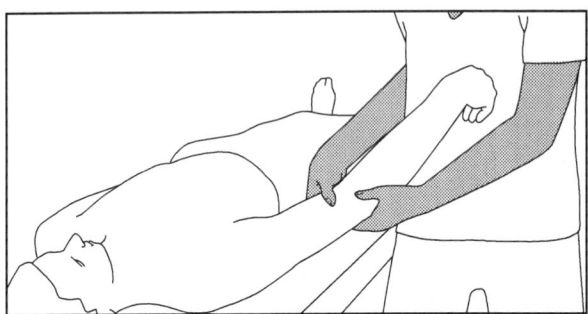

shoulder joint, avoiding traction to the elbow and forearm. It is for this reason that you need to find a way to clasp the arm above the elbow joint. You may find that it helps if your client positions their hand on the inside of your own arm, as if holding your tricep, or for you to hold the arm with the elbow flexed. Whichever handhold you settle on, it is important that you avoid tractioning the elbow: you want your 'pull' to be focused more proximally, at the shoulder joint. Practice with different handholds until both you and the client feel comfortable.

Question: Why should I avoid tractioning the elbow?

When you traction the upper limb, force is transmitted through the soft tissues (skin, fascia, muscle, tendons, ligaments, nerves, blood vessels, etc.). **If you hold the upper limb at the arm** (that is, the bicep/tricep region) and apply gentle traction, the force of this gentle stretch is transmitted through the shoulder, and through the soft tissues connecting the shoulder to the neck. **If you hold the limb below the elbow** (at the forearm region), this force is transmitted through the soft tissues of the elbow, through the arm, and then through the shoulder and neck, with decreasing stretch being felt in the shoulder and neck. **If you hold the upper limb by the hand**, the force of the stretch is transmitted through the wrist, forearm, elbow, arm, shoulder and finally some of the soft tissues of the neck. There are two reasons for placing your hands superior to the elbow. The first is that you want the focus of the stretch to be in the soft tissues of the shoulder and the neck. Holding the limb superior to the elbow achieves this. The second, is to avoid tractioning the elbow joint itself, or indeed any of the tissues distal to this, because even though the force you apply is *extremely* gentle with this stretch, in many people it can feel uncomfortable, especially where there is tension in tissues of the upper limb. There *are* techniques which involve handholds distal to the elbow, but for the technique being described here, try your best to hold the limb so that your stretch is focused on the shoulder and neck regions only.

Tip: With a colleague, practice holding each other's arm at the wrist, at the forearm, and then as shown below, and compare how it feels when you are the recipient of the stretch as it is performed with each of the different hand-holds.

Step 2 Keeping the client's arm close to their body, apply *gentle* traction and sustain this. Maintain your position. Tell yourself to relax. Discourage your client from talking but, of course, encourage them to let you know if they feel uncomfortable and stop the traction if they report discomfort. As you maintain the traction, see if you can get a sense of the client relaxing. Can you

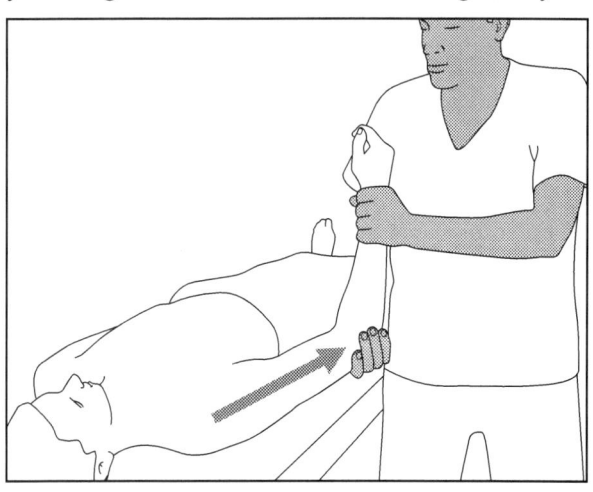

also get a sense of the tissues of the arm and
shoulder 'releasing'? Relaxation and release may
take a little time as the client settles into the
position, acclimatizes to the technique, and allows
themselves to 'let go'.

Step 3 For some clients, this very simple shoulder
stretch may be enough to provide some relief for a
stiff neck, as the soft tissues joining both
structures gradually release. However, some
subjects may get more benefit if they *slowly* turn
their head away from you—simply rolling it to the
opposite direction only as far as they feel
comfortable—once you are in position and have
applied the stretch. It is important that you apply
traction *first*, before the client turns their head
away from you. In this way it is the client who is
in control of how far they rotate, and therefore in
control of how much tension is placed on the soft
tissues of their neck and shoulder. Can you see
how, if the client were to rotate *before* you applied
traction, it would be you, the therapist, who was in
control of the stretch? If you were to perform the
stretch that way, with the client turning their head
first, before you applied traction, you could
potentially stress the tissues too much.

Step 4 After a couple of minutes, gently release both positions: encourage the client to return their head to neutral (if they had rotated it away from you), and relax the traction. Gently return the client's arm to rest on the treatment couch and repeat the technique on the opposite arm.

Question: Is this technique the same as a myofascial release (MFR) arm pull?

No, when performing a myofascial release arm pull you hold the hand and wrist, with slight supination of the forearm. Myofascial release arm pulls can be very beneficial and it is worth training in MFR if this is something that interests you.

TIP 3 TWO TECHNIQUES USING A TOWEL TO INCREASE RANGE OF MOVEMENT

Here is the first of two very gentle techniques that employ the use of a towel to increase range of movement in the neck. For each technique you will find it helpful to use a towel that is not too thick, about the size of a hand towel.

Technique 1
Position your client in the supine position with the towel beneath their head. When they are comfortable, grasp each end of the towel as shown and use it to gently move the client's head from side to side, letting the head roll one way and then the other. Be sure to move the head *slowly*.

Tip: Avoid the temptation to lift the head from the couch because when the head is lifted, some clients have an instinctive tendency to tense their neck muscles. Many clients feel safer, and are therefore more able to relax, when they can feel their head supported by the couch.

The advantage of this technique is that it facilitates rotation without you having to touch the client's head and face with your hands. Some clients enjoy receiving the sensation of passive neck rotation but dislike having oily hands on their face or hair. It is worth experiencing this technique for yourself to help determine what speed of motion left-to-right and right-to-left feels most appropriate.

Question: Are there any clients for whom this movement is contraindicated?

For most of the clients who could receive neck massage, this technique is safe. However, as it involves a rotatory movement, be cautious when using this technique with clients suffering inner ear disorders such as Ménière's disease.

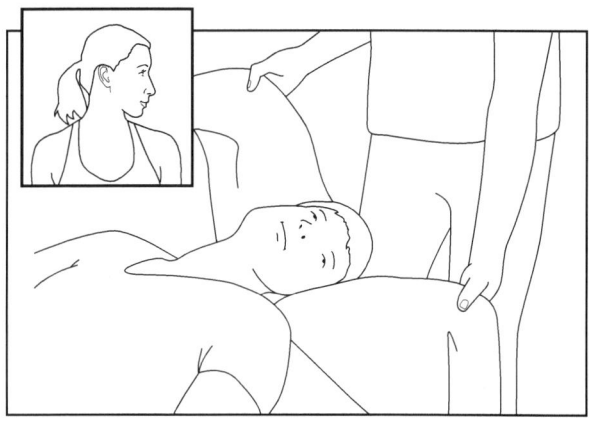

Technique 2

You can modify the previous tip so that instead of
facilitating rotation, you facilitate lateral flexion of
the neck. To do this, simply alter the position into
which you take the head, taking care to get
feedback from the client because, as you lengthen
and perhaps stretch one side of the neck, you
passively compress the opposite side of the neck.

Tip: Only keep the neck in lateral flexion for a
short time because muscles on the shortened side
sometimes cramp.

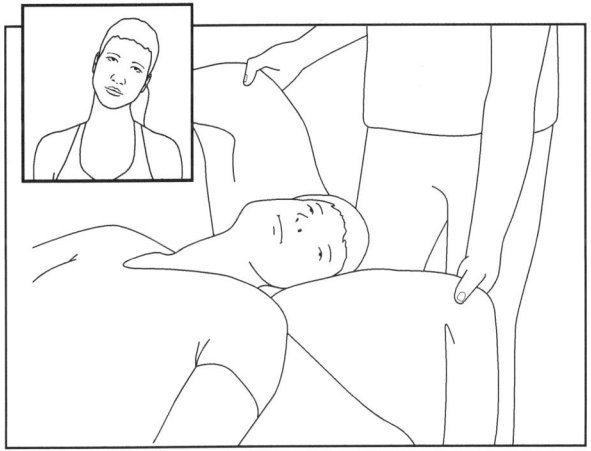

TIP 4 RELEASING THE POSTERIOR NECK TISSUES WITH GENTLE PASSIVE STRETCH

In their excellent book, *The Myofascial Release Manual*, Manheim and Lavette describe how to release tension in the soft tissues of the back of the neck in a manner with which you may not yet be familiar: myofascial release. If you are reading this as a massage therapist, it is important to realize that the technique described in this tip should be performed without the application of a massage medium. The technique is very gentle, yet even so, use of oil or wax would make it difficult for your fingertips to get enough purchase on the skin to facilitate the relaxation in tissues. Therefore when practicing this technique, do so without any oil or wax, but on dry skin only.

Step 1 With your client in the supine position, make sure you too are comfortable at the head of the couch. Once you have performed this technique once, you will have a better idea of whether or not you need to change your treatment position, from standing to sitting for example.

Manheim, C.J. and Lavett, D.K., 1989. *The Myofascial Release Manual*. New Jersey: Slack Incorporated.

Manheim and Lavette suggest that you position your client so that you have adequate support for your elbows on the treatment couch.

Step 2 Begin by gently cradling the client's head, gaining their confidence and encouraging them to relax. Start to stroke the back of the neck, slowly, and when you are ready choose one of the four handholds on the next page.

Step 3 Apply very *gentle*, sustained traction, just enough for you to feel some resistance in the tissues. Hold this position and wait. Wait until you sense the tissues release. Once you feel this release, either stop, or apply gentle traction again.

Tip: Practice using each of the four handholds, perhaps on different subjects, and decide with which hand position you feel most comfortable. You could practice all four handholds on the same person, but remember, you don't want to fatigue your client by overtreating them. You are likely to discover that, as with other techniques, given the variety of human anatomy, different handholds suit different clients.

Alternative handholds

a) Cupping the head at the base of the skull with one hand and applying slight overpressure with the other

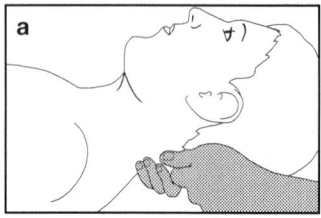

b) Cupping the base of the skull with both hands

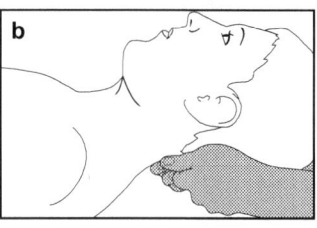

c) Cupping the base of the skull with one hand and placing the other on the client's shoulder.

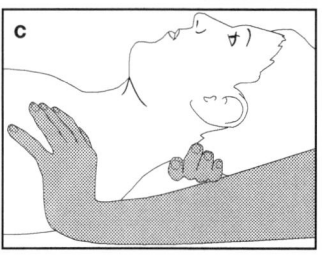

d) One hand on the client's sternum, against their skin, and the other hand cupping the base of the skull. (You may feel that this is inappropriate for some clients.)

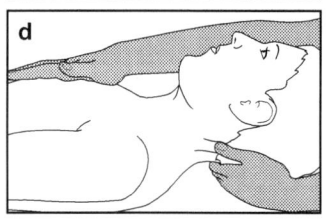

TIP 5 BE CAREFUL WITH OVERPRESSURE IN NECK FLEXION

A better understanding of anatomy can help you to become a better therapist. A good example of how knowing your anatomy can help inform your treatment is when you consider the form and function of the top two cervical vertebrae. C1 and C2—atlas and axis as they are called— have facet joints orientated at a different angle to the facet joints of other cervical vertebrae. In vertebrae C3 to C7 the facet joints are slanted at an angle. The facet joints between atlas and axis are also slanted, but to a lesser degree.

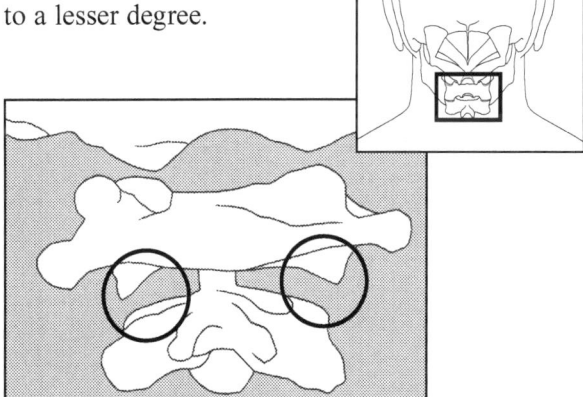

Relatively speaking, the atlanto-axial facet joints are orientated more horizontally than the facet joints in the rest of the cervical spine. So how does that information help inform our practice?

Well, flexion of the head and neck with overpressure is often performed to stretch the soft tissues on the back of the neck. Yet in flexion, the facet joints of the atlas and axis bones are compressed. Flexion with overpressure, as is common in neck flexion stretches, may put excessive strain on the facet joints between these top two cervical vertebrae. This is not a problem in most healthy individuals, but may pose a risk when treating clients with osteoporosis or those who have a pathology affecting their facet joints. In such cases, there is a good argument for avoiding both active and passive stretches involving overpressure in flexion of the head and neck. Alternative stretches may be safer. The next tip describes a method for stretching the posterior neck tissues *without* flexion.

TIP 6 USING A TOWEL TO FACILITATE A PASSIVE NECK STRETCH

For those clients who enjoy the sensation of a slightly stronger stretch than those described in *Tip 4* (pp.128-130), this next technique may prove useful. It is easy to perform but note, the strength of the stretch as perceived by the client is partially influenced by how you hold the towel and the height of your treatment couch.

Step 1 Position your client in the supine position with a small hand towel beneath their head. Make sure they have removed any earrings. Check the position of the towel. It should be placed so that when you lift it, it hooks nicely into the occipital bone, the base of the skull. Grasp the towel as close to your client's face as possible. This is important for if you grasp the towel too far away from the face, the stretch feels quite different to receive and instead of gentle traction you end up tilting the head back a little into extension.

Step 2 Slowly and carefully start to bring your arms toward you, gently stretching the muscles of the posterior neck.

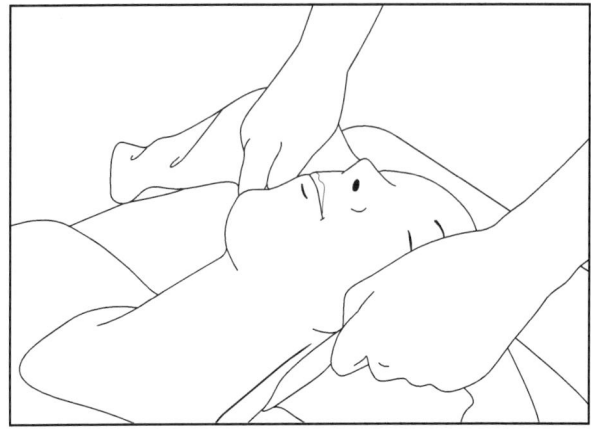

Tip: One trick is to use the very edge of the towel, rather than a towel edge that has been folded over, as this gives a better 'hook' into the occiput.

Tip: Your client cannot hear you when receiving this stretch as the towel covers their ears. It is therefore useful to agree beforehand on a simple signal to indicate if the stretch feels too strong and the client wishes you to stop. One such signal is simply for them to raise their hand.

TIP 7   CHANGING THE TREATMENT POSITION

One of the things you might consider in order to provide variety for both yourself and for your clients, and as an experiment when working with clients with whom you are not progressing as quickly as you would like, is to change the position in which the client has been receiving treatment. Consider changing from prone to supine, or from supine to seated, or from seated to side lying, for example. *Tips 8, 9, 10* and *11* provide ideas on how you might utilize different treatment positions to your advantage. To begin, here is a summary of the advantages and disadvantages of each position.

PRONE	
Advantages	**Disadvantages**
• Allows easy access to the back of the neck. • Tissues of the back of the neck can be seen and assessed visually, facilitating treatment to muscles such as levator scapulae, trapezius, paraspinals.	• Tissues of the anterior neck cannot safely be treated; tissues on the side of the neck may be more difficult to treat in this position. • Not always suitable for clients who feel claustrophobic.

| PRONE (CONTINUED) ||
Advantages	Disadvantages
• Makes linking the back of the neck to the shoulders and thorax easy using massage strokes. • The therapist can stand at the head or at the side of the treatment couch. • Can be a useful position when treating clients who are severely kyphotic. • Can be useful when needing to treat the base of the occiput, insertion of sternocleidomastoid or the back of the head.	• Communication is more difficult: Clients cannot always hear the therapist in this position; therapists cannot always hear the client. • Can make treating clients with a very lordotic neck or kinked neck difficult, unless the client is able to chin tuck comfortably. • Can be uncomfortable for clients with low back problems unless a pillow is placed beneath the stomach. • Is not appropriate for clients in later stages of pregnancy, or clients whose anterior is affected by discomfort, recent injury, or surgery (e.g., abdominal bloating, anterior knee pain, mastectomy). • Some clients dislike the temporary mark left on the face or forehead from the face cradle. • Resting in the prone position too long, some clients discover their nose starts to run.

SUPINE	
Advantages	**Disadvantages**
• Tissues of the anterior and side of the neck are easy to access, facilitating treatment to scalenes and sternocleidomastoid. • Although the posterior neck tissues cannot be seen, they can be palpated in this position and are sometimes easier to palpate this way owing to the decrease in tone resulting from a relaxed head position. • Can be very useful when treating clients who cannot comfortably lie prone. • Makes linking the front and sides of the neck to the chest easy using massage strokes. • Can be a useful position when there needs to be an ongoing dialogue between the client and the therapist.	• May be more difficult to access tissues of the posterior neck. • Posterior neck tissues cannot be seen. • May be uncomfortable for clients with an exaggerated kyphotic curve. • Can be uncomfortable for clients with lumber problems unless they rest with hips and knees flexed or a bolster beneath their knees. • Is contraindicated in later stages of pregnancy.

SIDE LYING

Advantages	Disadvantages
• Makes the side of the neck that is uppermost easy to access. • Can be very useful when treating clients who cannot easily or safely lie prone or supine, such as in later stages of pregnancy. • Tissues can easily be passively shortened or passively lengthened in this position, facilitating access to deeper structures. • Makes linking the side of the neck to the shoulder easy using massage strokes.	• The client has to swap sides during treatment and this can interrupt the flow of the session. • Can be difficult for the client to find a comfortable position for the arm on which they are resting. • May not be suitable for clients with shoulder problems who could find resting on their shoulder painful.

SEATED	
Advantages	**Disadvantages**
• Is a very useful treatment position for when you want the client to be more engaged with the treatment they are receiving, or, when it is important for there to be an ongoing dialogue. • Can be very useful when treating clients who cannot easily or safely lie prone or supine, such as in later stages of pregnancy. • Facilitates access to the front, sides and to the back of the neck.	• The client may be less relaxed than in a lying position. • Tissues of the neck are under more tension when the client is seated than in other treatment positions. • Unless a face cradle is available, there is an increase in tone in muscles of the neck in the seated position as these work to support the head, even when the client attempts to relax.

TIP 8 FIVE WAYS TO ACCESS THE NECK IN THE PRONE POSITION

1. Chin tuck

One of the ways you can gain better access to the back of the neck is to ask your client to tuck in their chin when they are resting in the prone position. By doing this they actively reposition their head into a more flexed position, thus lengthening the tissues on the posterior of the neck and helping to slightly gap the vertebrae posteriorly. This is especially helpful when treating clients with an excessively lordotic neck, a kinked neck, or with a dowager's hump—a fatty overgrowth of tissue that makes accessing the

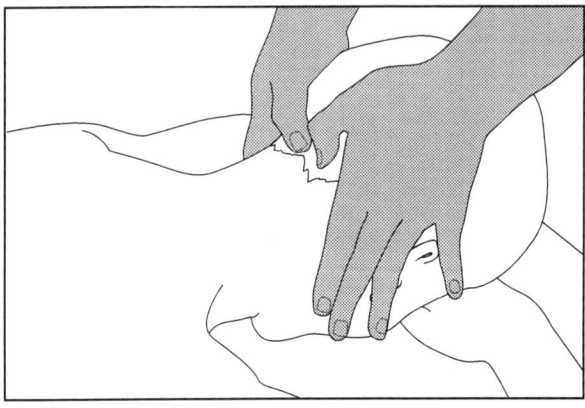

tissues of the posterior neck tricky at times. Clients may choose to do the chin tuck while resting with their face in a face hole or face cradle, or, they may chose simply to rest their forehead on their hands. Whichever method they choose, this repositioning helps you gain access to the posterior neck, but remember that in this chin tuck position the posterior neck tissues are lengthened and under slightly more tension than when a client rests prone.

2. Using a sponge to passively retract scapulae

When a client rests prone, without the aid of any supports, their shoulders fall naturally into protraction. Placing a large sponge, a small rolled up towel, or a tiny cushion beneath the client's shoulder as they rest in the prone position has the effect of passively retracting the scapula and in so doing passively shortens some of the tissues linking the neck and shoulder. Passively shortening these tissue can help you to gain access to deeper tissues. To prove this for yourself, try both positions. Have your client lie face down in the prone position, their shoulders allowed to fall forward, into protraction. Massage the upper fibers of trapezius. How does this muscle feel to you? Is it malleable yet quite firm? Next, reposition your client by gently inserting a bath sponge, for example, beneath one of their shoulders. Now massage the upper trapezius. Can you feel how much softer the tissues feel now they have been passively shortened? See if you can palpate more deeply, identifying levator scapalae, the strap-like muscle running from the transverse processes of

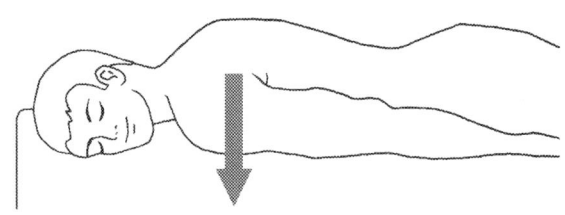

Without support

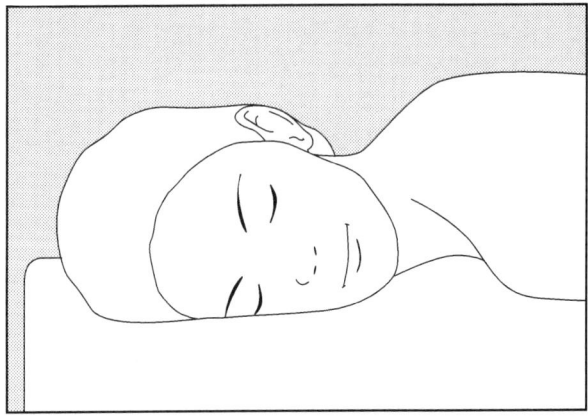

the top three to four cervical vertebrae and
inserting onto the superior angle of the scapula.
Can you identify this muscle which is often
lengthened and feels 'twangy'?

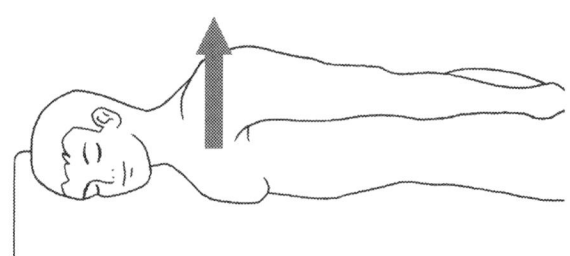

With support

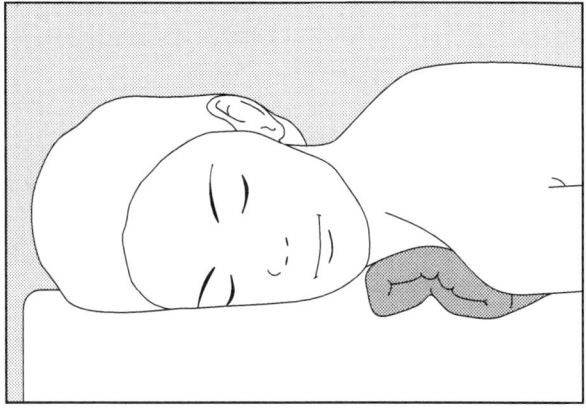

3. Using your thigh for support

If you don't have access to a support such as a towel or large sponge, you can position yourself as shown and passively abduct the arm, retracting the scapula. Sit on the edge of the treatment couch and gently support the client's arm in abduction, allowing it to rest on your thigh. You may feel that this is not an appropriate treatment position for all clients.

Tip: Avoid drawing the client's shoulder into too much horizontal extension as this can cause an uncomfortable stretch on the anterior of the shoulder. Some clients experience temporary pins and needles in their fingers due to temporary compression of nerves or vascular structures in the arm.

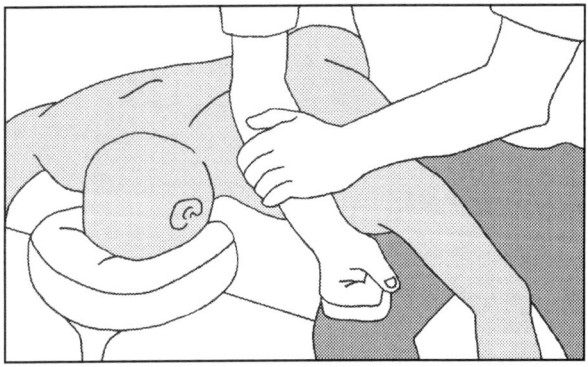

4. Working with the shoulder elevated

Another position you could try if you haven't already, is to position the client with their shoulder in elevation. Whilst this passively shortens the soft tissues crossing the neck and shoulder joints, the disadvantage is that this position can trigger cramping or feelings of impingement in the supraspinatus muscle of some clients. This is because muscles sometimes cramp when passively shortened. It would therefore not be appropriate when treating someone with supraspinatus tendinosis, or a torticollis.

Tip: This position also facilitates palpation of the scalenes on the anterior neck.

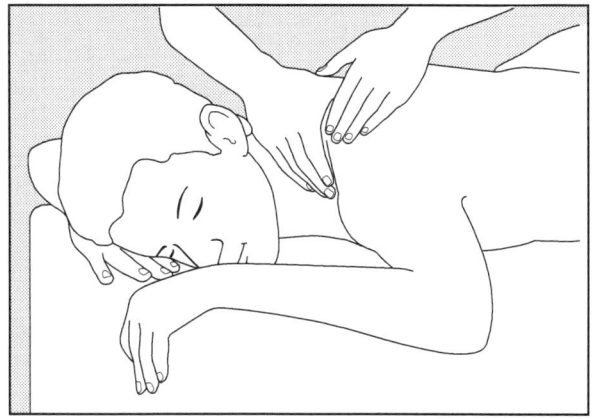

5. Opening up the posterior region by increasing flexion

Many therapists choose to use a treatment couch with an adjustable face cradle. Providing that the client is comfortable, you can experiment with facilitating varying degrees of neck flexion, thus facilitating better access to the back of the neck. This is helpful when working with clients who are very kyphotic, those who are very overweight and who may have rather large necks, or those with a dowager's hump.

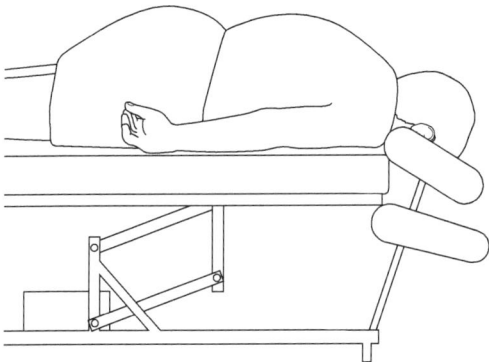

On the next two pages is a table comparing the advantages and disadvantages of each of the five ways to access the neck in the prone position. Once you have had a chance to experiment, add your own notes. Do you agree or disagree with any of these points? What could you add?

Advantages	Disadvantages
ACTIVE OR PASSIVE CHIN TUCK	
• Enables access to posterior neck tissues. • Good for treating clients with short necks or with a lot of fat in the neck region.	• Some clients feel squashed or claustrophobic. • If performed actively, difficult to maintain position for long periods without fatigue.
PASSIVE SCAPULA RETRACTION WITH SPONGE	
• Facilitates access to deeper structures such as levator scapulae.	• Some clients feel uncomfortable with one shoulder retracted. • Uncomfortable for clients with tight anterior shoulder muscles.
PASSIVE SCAPULA RETRACTION USING THIGH	
• Facilitates access to deeper structures such as levator scapulae. • Therapist does not need any extra equipment to bring about the retraction.	• May be considered too intimate a position for some therapists/clients. • An uncomfortable treatment position for some therapists. • Some clients feel uncomfortable having one shoulder passively retracted in this way. • Uncomfortable for clients with tight anterior shoulder muscles.

Advantages	Disadvantages
POSITION 4. PASSIVE SCAPULA ELEVATION	
• Facilitates access to deeper structures such as levator scapulae.	• Can trigger temporary spasm in upper fibers of trapezius and levator scapulae in some cases. • Not appropriate for treatment of shoulder impingement syndromes.
POSITION 5. PASSIVE NECK FLEXION	
• Enables access to posterior neck tissues. • Good for treating clients with short necks or with a lot of fat in the neck region.	• Not all clients feel comfortable with their head in this slight downward position. • Addition of a face cradle makes it harder to access lower regions of the back from the head of the couch (e.g., with effleurage) when incorporating neck treatments into a back massage.

TIP 9 FIVE TREATMENT TECHNIQUES WITH YOUR CLIENT IN THE PRONE POSITION

1. Pulling into the occiput

Useful to help lengthen posterior neck tissues as you drag your fingers towards you, bringing about gentle traction on the skin, which sometimes draws the head into slight flexion. Or, alternatively, simply cradle your fingers beneath the occiput and wait to sense the subtle changes in pliability of the tissues against your fingertips.

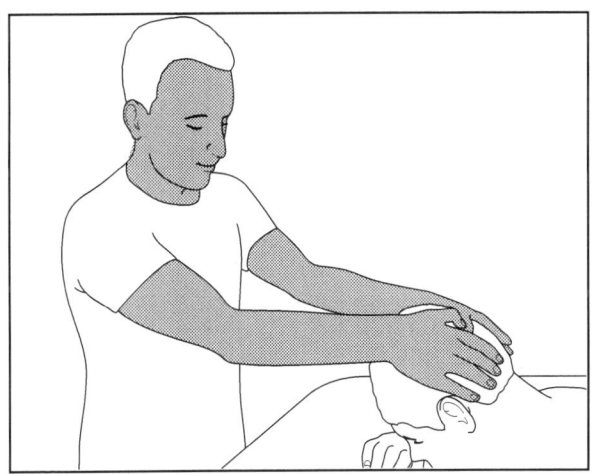

2. Gentle gripping of posterior neck muscles

In the prone position it is easy to gently grip the tissues of the back of the neck and ever so gently pull them upwards, away from the spine. This can feel very relaxing providing you avoid pinching the skin too tightly.

Experiment with different massage mediums. Notice that if you use oil it can be difficult to get a purchase on the muscles in order to pull them gently towards you. One tip is to practice without any massage medium at all. How does your client feel if you simply pull and hold the tissues? Does it matter where you stand in relation to your subject?

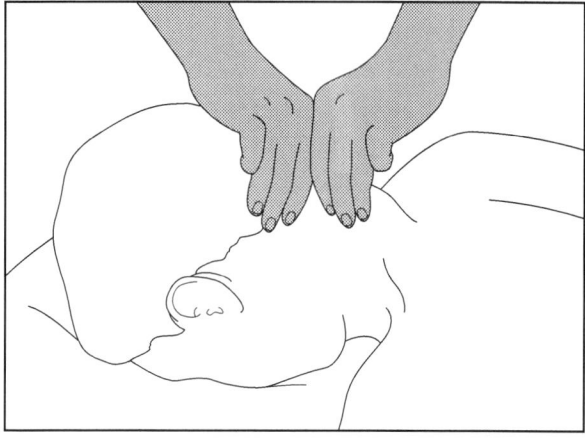

3. Gentle static pressures to trigger spots

If you are able to identify a trigger spot it can be relieved with gentle, static pressure. If using your thumbs as shown below, be careful where you position your fingers. It can be tempting to rest them on the sides of the client's neck and jaw as shown below, but this can feel unpleasant for some clients. Note that if you are on a trigger spot, discomfort should resolve within about 60 seconds. If the spot continues to be painful, release your pressure. Be cautious when treating trigger points of clients with known neck pathologies, and avoid pressure to the vertebrae in osteoporotic subjects.

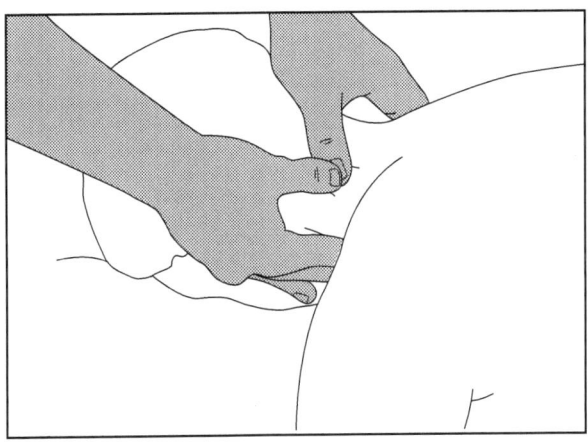

152 Perhaps you have located a trigger point in the trapezius. Such points are easily treated in the prone position. You could treat the point as shown here, or you could treat it with the shoulder in passive retraction as shown in *Tip 8* (pp.145). As you apply gentle pressure to the trigger spot, discomfort should start to dissipate. Avoid pressing too hard. Remember the theme of *Neck Treatment Tips* is 'less is more'.

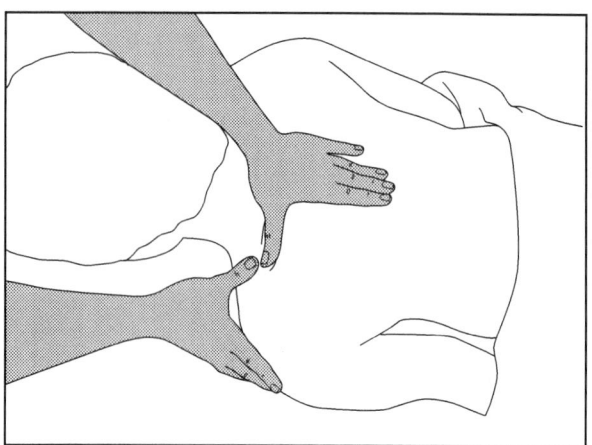

4. Short, caudal strokes

Small, longitudinal strokes can be applied from the client's head to the base of their neck (i.e. in caudal direction).

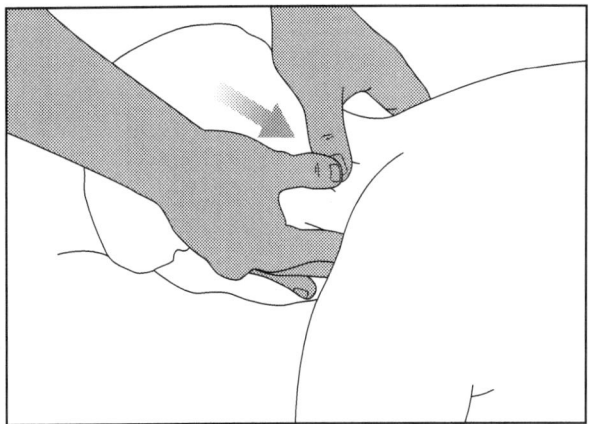

When treating in this way, be careful with the positioning of your fingers. Avoid gripping the sides of the neck at the same time you are stroking downward, toward the shoulders; avoid using your fingers for leverage when applying thumb pressure. It may be necessary to flex your fingers, especially if you have large hands or when treating a client with a small neck. Compare stroking the neck with reinforced thumbs to stroking with alternate thumbs. Which feels best for you?

5. Gentle transverse stretch using digital pressure

Alternatively, reinforce one of your fingers as shown here, either to apply gentle, static pressure to a trigger point, or to gently roll the skin and tissues transversely. Remember, you do not necessarily need to 'rub' the tissues back and forth. This can irritate a point of discomfort rather than alleviate it. Instead, practice gently pushing the tissues away from you, allow for there to be a little traction on the skin, and wait to see if you can feel the tissues 'creep' and release.

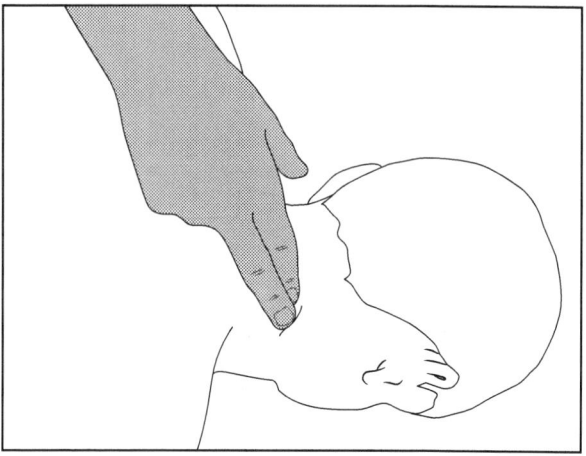

The table on the next page summarizes uses for these five prone-position techniques.

Uses of each technique

1. Pulling into the occiput:
- Acclimatizing the client to your touch
- Starting and ending a treatment

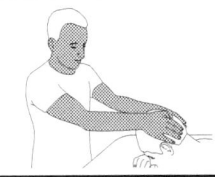

2. Gentle gripping:
- Passively stretching neck extensor muscles and fascia without moving joints of the neck
- Palpating for trigger spots.

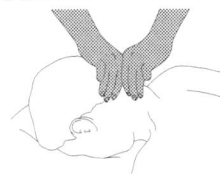

3. Static pressures:
- Alleviation of trigger points in neck extensor muscles with neck muscles relaxed

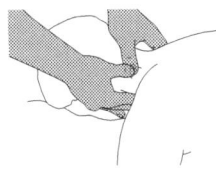

4. Short, caudal strokes:
- Soothing tissues after deactivation of trigger points
- Applying localized longitudinal stretch to neck extensor tissues

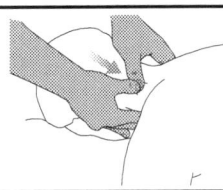

5. Transverse stretch:
- Passively stretching neck extensor muscles without moving cervical joints
- Localizing stretch of tissues to a specific spot

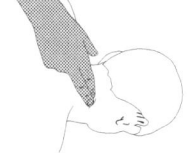

TIP 10 TIPS FOR TREATING THE NECK IN THE SUPINE POSITION

Treating clients in the supine position gives you the opportunity to treat all regions of the neck, and later tips provide specific ideas for how to treat scalenes, sternocleidomastoid and occipitals in this position. Neck retractions, an exercise you will find described in *Part 3, Tip 7* (p.258) can sometimes work better with the client in this position.

Some techniques work best when you remove the pillow, yet some clients may feel more comfortable with a neck support in the form of a small rolled up towel, especially if they have an increased cervical lordosis. Conversely, you may wish to facilitate a decrease in such a lordosis by placing a small towel beneath the head.

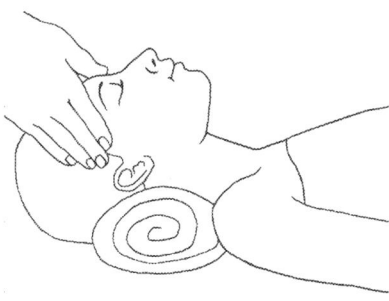

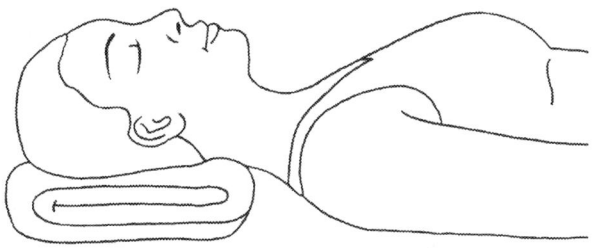

When a client is supine their neck is in a neutral position. Some clients may feel more comfortable if they are allowed to rest in slight neck flexion, although this can make treatment more difficult for you, and you may find that you need to lower your treatment couch considerably.

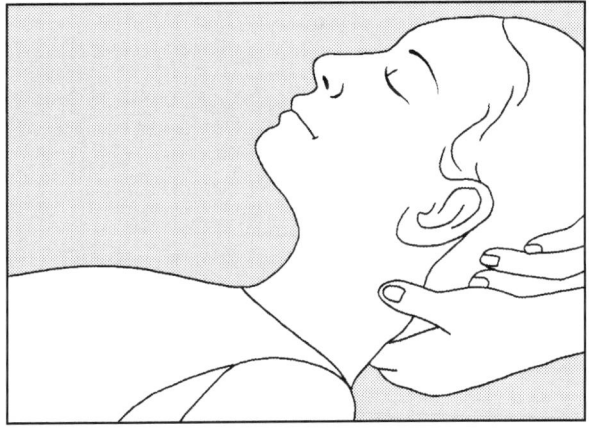

The supine position enables you to gently lift and cradle the head, to turn it gently side to side, something many clients find very soothing.

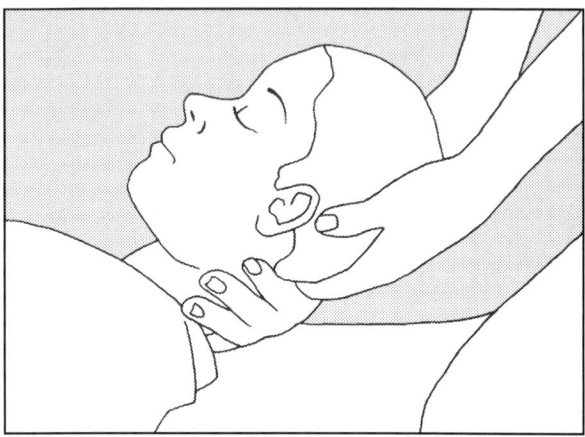

Tip: Experiment by role playing with a colleague. When playing the therapist, give the instruction to 'relax and let go' while holding the head as shown here. Then say, 'again, relax and let go'. See if you can identify the point at which 'client' relaxes both on the first instruction and on the second.

Techniques you can use with your client in the
supine position include passive depression of the
shoulders unilaterally or bilaterally (a), gentle
stroking of the neck (b), and passive neck stretches
such as the one shown overleaf, with the head and
neck being taken gently into lateral flexion (c).

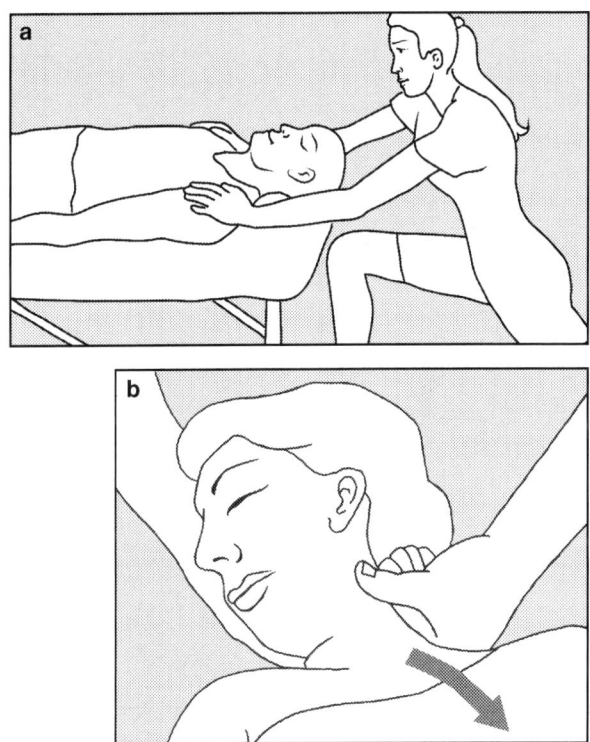

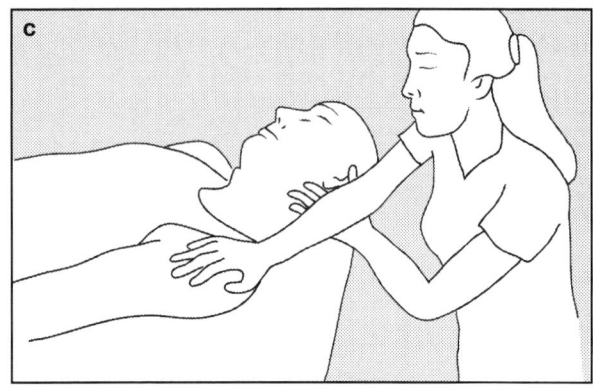

Additional techniques in supine

In addition to these last three techniques, at the beginning of *Neck Treatment Tips* you learned how gentle shoulder traction could enhance a neck stretch, and were introduced to three neck stretches using a towel with your client in the supine position (one rotatory, one lateral and one cephelad). You also learned that useful myofascial stretches can be applied with a client in supine. Later you will learn how to release suboccipital muscles using your fingertips and how to treat sternocleidomastoid and scalenes, some of the techniques for which are applied in supine. Once you are familiar with these techniques, you could return to the chart on the next three pages and tick those techniques you have tried and circle those you want to practice again.

Technique	1	2	3
1. Gentle shoulder traction 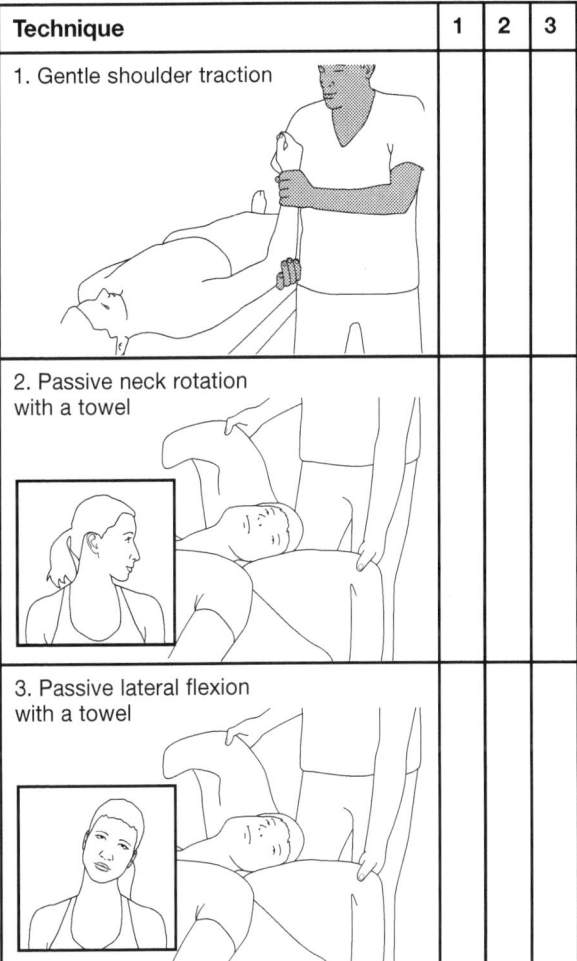			
2. Passive neck rotation with a towel			
3. Passive lateral flexion with a towel			

Technique	1	2	3
4. Passive (cephelad) stretch using a towel			
5. Myofascial release of tissues			
6. Fingertips to suboccipitals			

Technique	1	2	3
7. Bilateral depression of shoulders			
8. Unilateral depression of shoulders			
9. Passive lateral stretch			

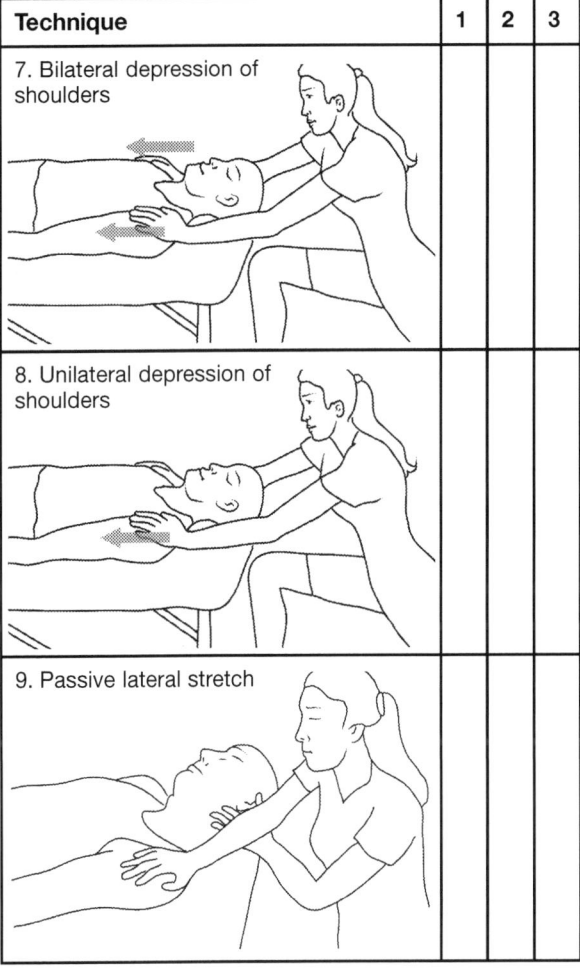

Technique	1	2	3
10. Longitudinal stroking 			
11. Gentle stretch to anterior tissues 			
12. Treating sternocleidomastoid 			

Technique	1	2	3
13. Treating scalenes			

Remember, these are only some of the techniques you could use. If you are a qualified therapist you may already be using some or many of these. If you are a student, there may be some you have not tried before. All of these can be interspersed with any techniques you are already using and with facial massage and massage to the anterior of the shoulders and to the chest.

An experiment in focus

Let's focus now on just two techniques, depression of the shoulders and compression of trigger points in the upper fibers of trapezius. As an exercise, practice with a colleague and spend five minutes on each side of the neck using only these two techniques. See if you can answer the following questions.

1. Depression of the shoulders:

- As you depress the shoulders one at a time, which feels easier to move, the left or the right shoulder? Does your subject sense any variation?
- Does it matter where you place your hands, on the top of the shoulder at the head of the humerus, or more anteriorly?
- Does it matter which part of your hand you use to apply the depression?
- How does it feel when you keep your palm in the same place but change the orientation of your fingers? Is this better or worse for your wrists as a therapist?
- How does it feel to slowly depress one shoulder and to hold it in gentle depression for 20 seconds?
- Finally, what happens if, as you gently depress the shoulder, your subject turns their head away from you? Do they experience a stretch or is this uncomfortable?

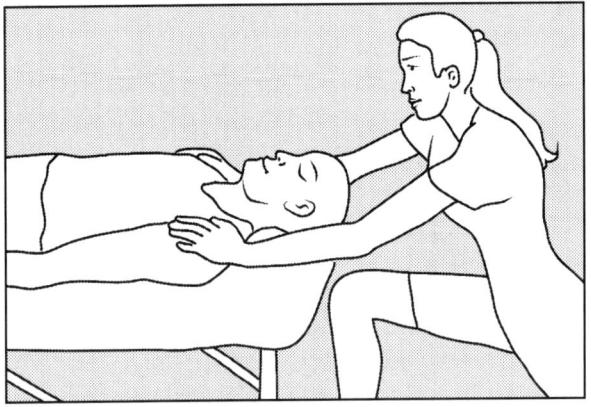

2. Applying gentle pressure to the trapezius on one side and palpating for trigger points:

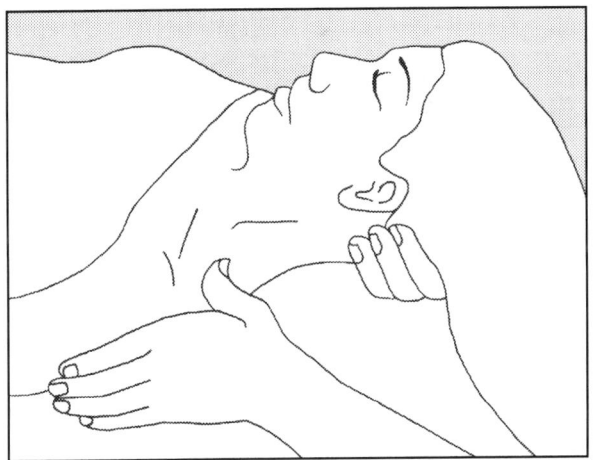

✹ What happens if you gently compress a point
and then use your other hand to slowly move
your subject's head away from the point,
tensioning the tissue. Is this relieving for your
client, or uncomfortable?

✹ How does your thumb feel, comfortable or
strained?

✹ Can you discover any trigger points? Where are
they? Are these lateral, close to the shoulder, or
are they closer to the neck? Or, do they fall in
the middle of these upper fibers of trapezius,
between the distal end of the clavicle and the
neck itself?

✹ How easy is it for you to compress the upper
fibers of trapezius in this position? Do you feel
that in order to access the trigger points properly
you need your client to be in a position other
than supine? Or can you access some of the
points in this position?

Note that there are no right or wrong answers to
these questions and you and your colleague may
have different experiences.

Use the table on the next page to record your
experiences

Shoulders feel equal to depress?	Yes/no
Best position to place hands	
Best part of hand to use	
Finger orientation?	
Sustained depression feels...	
Sustained shoulder depression with active head movement	
Location of trigger points	
Compression of triggers with active head movement	
Thumb pain	Yes/no

TIP 11 TIPS FOR TREATING THE NECK IN THE SIDE LYING POSITION

Experimenting with a pillow

This position can be useful in helping to 'open up' the neck region, providing access to the lateral side of neck. It requires some experimentation to discover the best use of a pillow with your client in the side lying position. Using a pillow can help make your client comfortable but can hinder access to the whole of the back of the neck. Sometimes it is difficult for a client to rest in this position without their arm and shoulder getting squashed. Also, not all clients can lie on both their left and right sides equally well. They may be more comfortable on one side than on the other so you cannot always expect to be able to treat both sides of the neck in this position. It is a useful position for treating pregnant clients or those for whom resting prone or supine is uncomfortable.

Tip: Remember that if your client is in the side lying position you may need to offer them a pillow or bolster for support between their legs or beneath the knee that is uppermost.

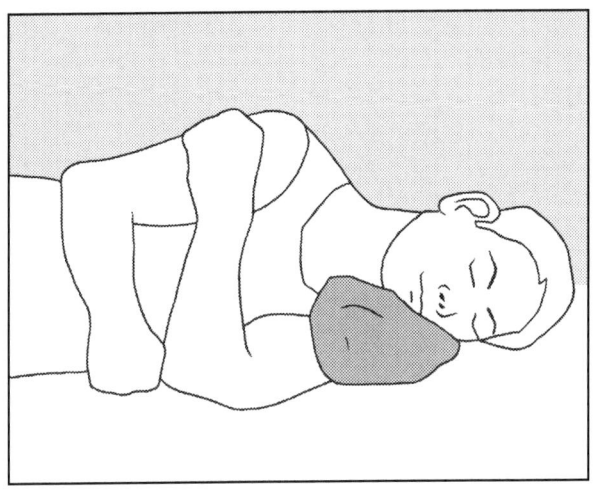

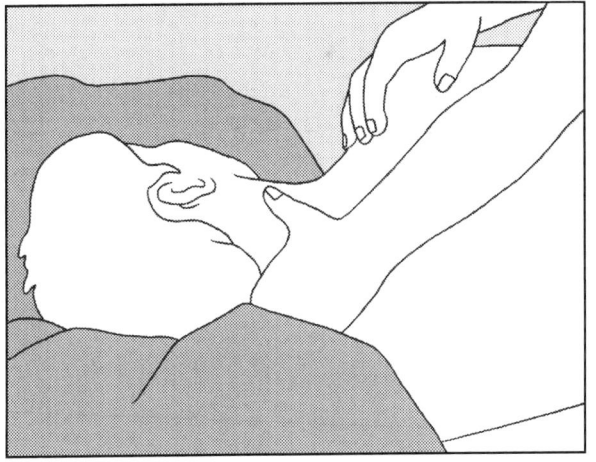

172 Passive abduction of the arm in side lying

Some therapists like to passively abduct the arm of their client as shown here. This has the effect of passively shortening some of the soft tissues spanning the shoulder and the neck and can therefore facilitate access to deeper structures. Not all clients are able to relax and 'give' you their arm in this manner.

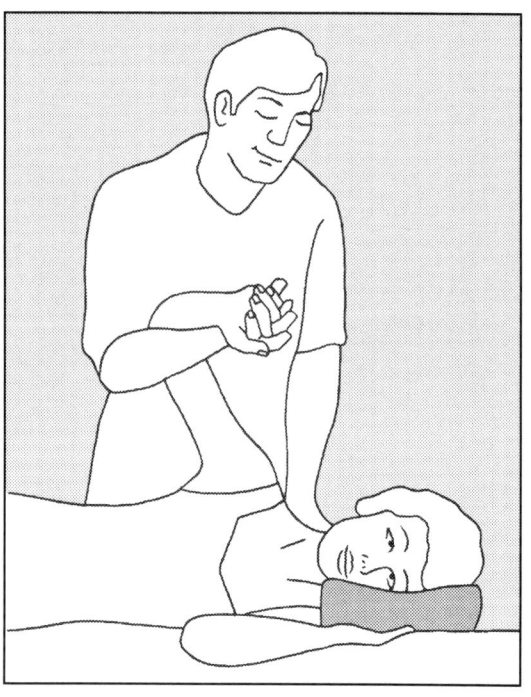

Stretching the neck in the side lying position

Try different handholds to see if you can apply a gentle stretch to the shoulder and neck muscles in the side lying position. Which method suits you best, standing at the head of the couch and gently depressing the client's shoulder, or hooking your arm in theirs to depress the shoulder that way?

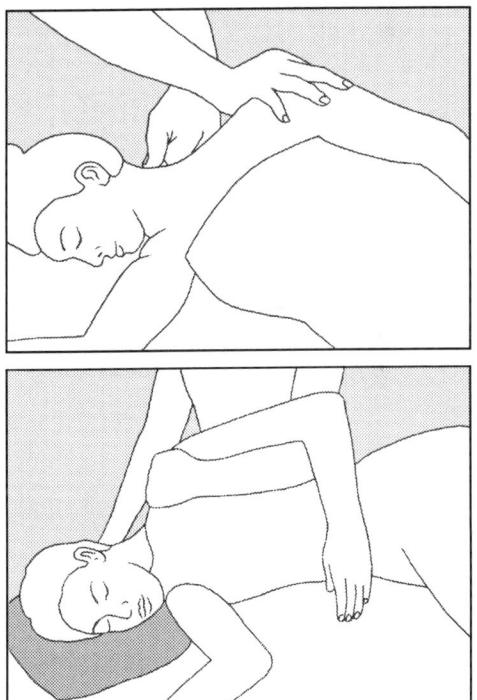

174 Forearm massage in side lying

In *Tip 8* (pp.141-143) you saw how changing the position of the shoulder in the prone position facilitated greater access to trapezius. Changing the position of the client entirely, from prone to three-quarter lying, is another way to help you access these tissues.

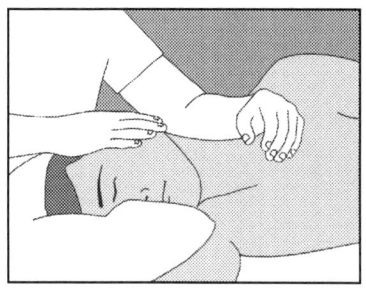

Sitting or kneeling at the head of the treatment couch, use your forearm to gently work into the tissues once you have warmed them up.

Be careful to keep your pressure light as you move over the transverse processes of the cervical vertebrae as too much pressure could cause bruising and discomfort. Deeper

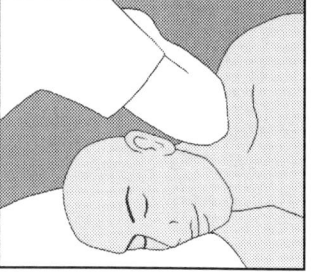

pressure can be used in the fleshy belly of the upper fibers of trapezius.

TIP 12 TIPS FOR TREATING THE NECK WITH YOUR CLIENT SEATED

Abduction of the arm in seated position

Practice palpating the upper part of trapezius with your client in a seated position. How do the tissues feel, are they soft and malleable or dense and stiff?

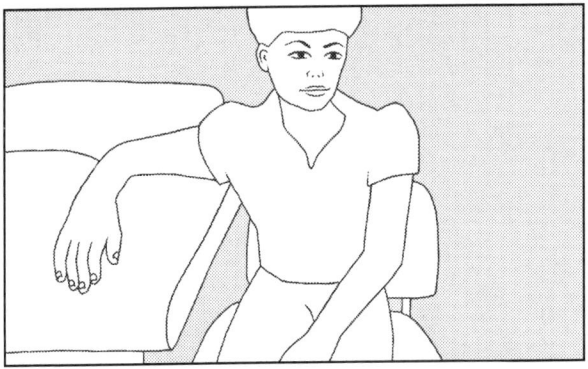

Next, find a way to passively abduct the shoulder of your client, perhaps using pillows. By placing the arm into passive abduction there is less tension on the upper part of trapezius and you have the advantage of being able to access underlying tissues more easily. In this altered position, palpate the upper fibers of trapezius again. How do the tissues feel, is there a difference?

Gripping trapezius with and without rotation

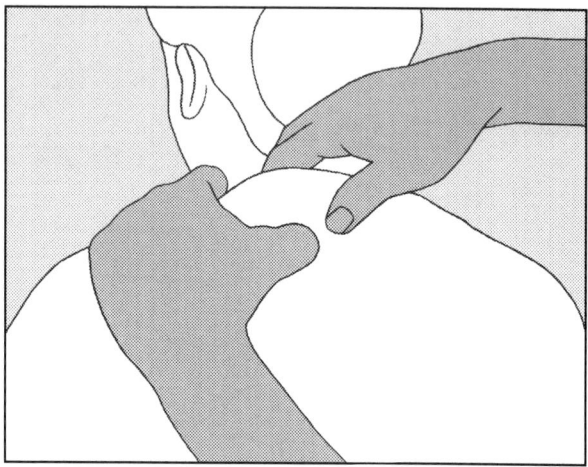

Another technique with your client seated, with or without passive arm abduction, is to gently grip the tissues of trapezius. This is not always possible, for, as you know, some clients have strong, dense tissues which are stiff and difficult to grip. However, sometimes simple gripping is all that is required to facilitate a reduction in tension.

An additional technique is to maintain a grip and to ask your client to gently turn their head away from you, bringing about a soft tissue stretch.

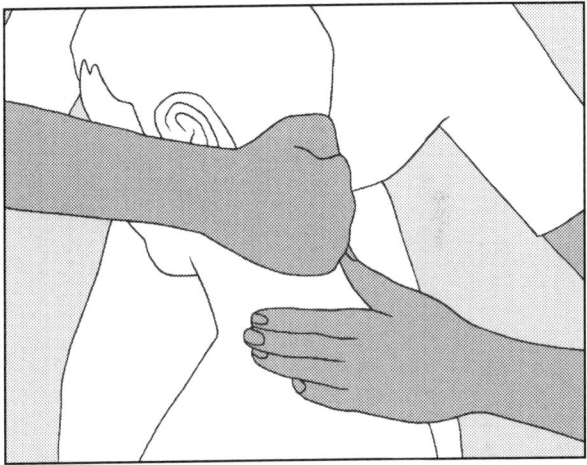

Gently stroking the tissues transversely away from the spine is soothing but requires you to support the client's head as shown and not all clients feel comfortable in this position. In sitting, the muscles of the neck are active as they try to support the head so this is not the most effective treatment position for reducing tension here. It is, however, useful when a client is unable, or does not wish, to lie on a couch to receive treatment.

Pressing into the occiput

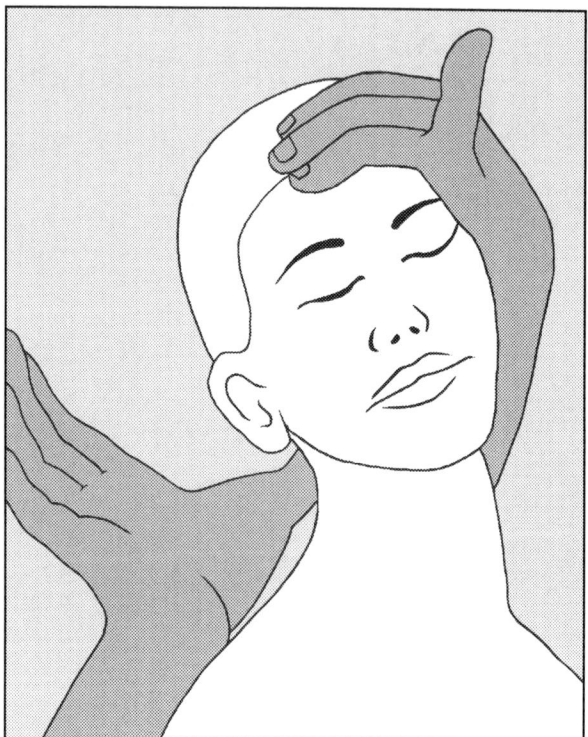

This can be helpful for applying gentle pressure to the suboccipital muscles. Taking the head gently back into extension helps to shorten the neck extensor muscles, facilitating greater access to deeper structures.

Linked fingers to 'pull off' soft tissues

Standing behind your subject, link your fingers, squeezing the soft tissues towards you. Keep your pressure light to avoid squashing tissues forcibly against the transverse processes of cervical vertebrae.

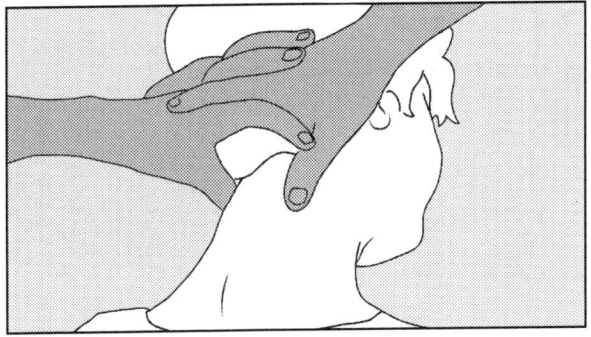

Alternatively, gently grip and draw the tissues toward you.

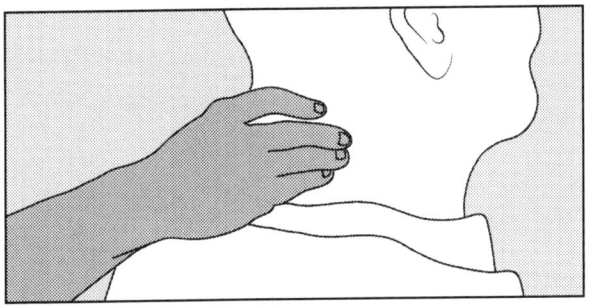

180 Use this chart and tick the boxes when you have practiced these seven techniques on three different clients.

Technique	1	2	3
1. Seated (without arm abduction)			
2. Seated with arm in abduction			
3. Gripping			

Technique	1	2	3
4. Gripping with active rotation			
5. Transverse strokes			
6. Gentle pressures to occiput			
7. Gentle gripping to back of neck			

TIP 13 TREATING SUBOCCIPITALS

In *Part 1: Neck Assessment Tips,* the importance
of the small occipital muscles was described in
Tip 19 (pp.80-81), and *Tip 20* (pp. 82-84) covered
how to palpate them. Here you will find some tips
on ways you might treat these muscles, using
various different treatment positions.

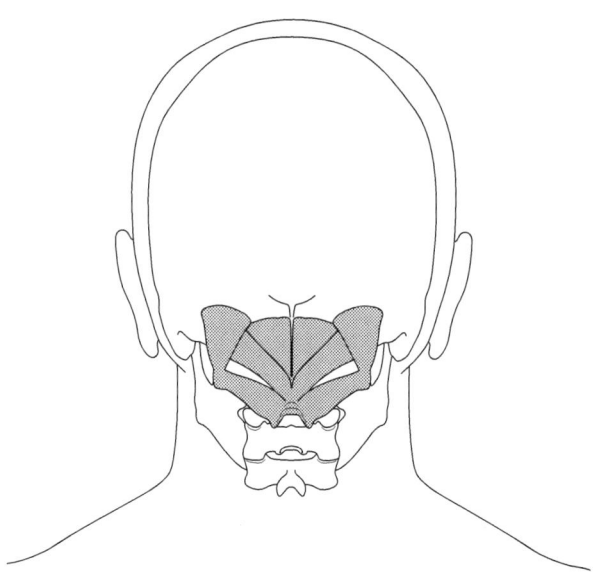

Prone

In the prone position, you can use your fingertips to gently massage the suboccipital area as you stand at the head of the couch, or you can simply rest your fingertips against the base of the skull and allow the gentlest of fingertip pressure to stimulate a decrease in tension. Sometimes, using your thumbs to gently press into the muscles on one side of the neck and then to gently push the skin from the occiput, down toward the base of the neck and toward the shoulders can be very soothing. Fingers or thumbs can be reinforced but often only very light touch is needed as you move from the hairline, down toward the lower cervical vertebrae.

Tip: As you practice either of these techniques— resting your fingertips or pushing the skin— ask yourself whether both left and right sides of the occipital region feel the same. If one feels different, in what way is it different? Is it more firm to palpate? More pliable? Less pliable? Do the tissues seem to move in the same manner as on the opposite side of the occiput? Can you identify any localized trigger points or do you feel that this region of the neck is too dense for you to identify trigger points through palpation?

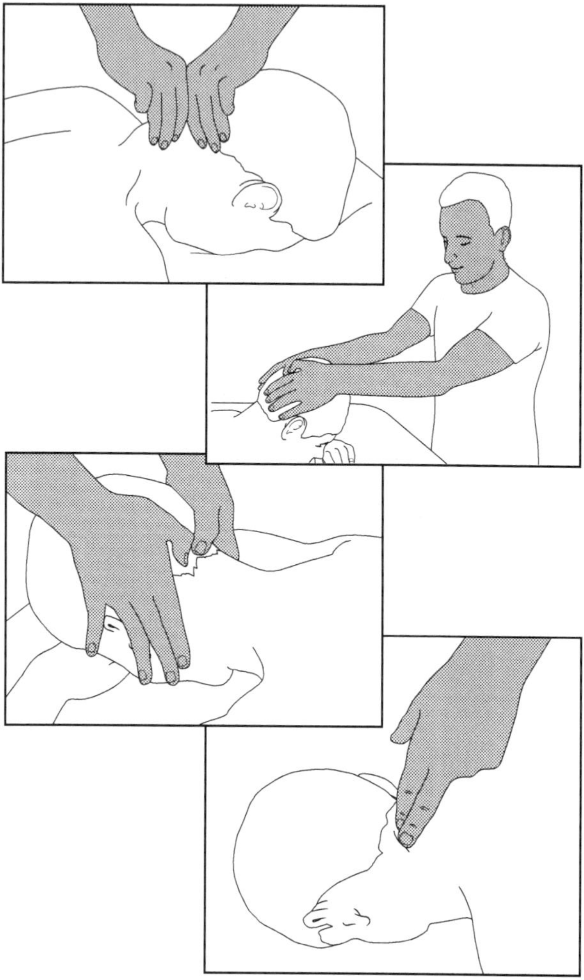

Supine

In the supine position, posterior neck muscles are relaxed, and palpation can sometimes be easier than when the client is prone. Working with a client supine, you have the opportunity to assess the suboccipital region for tenderness and trigger points and to use the weight of the client's head to assist in the treatment.

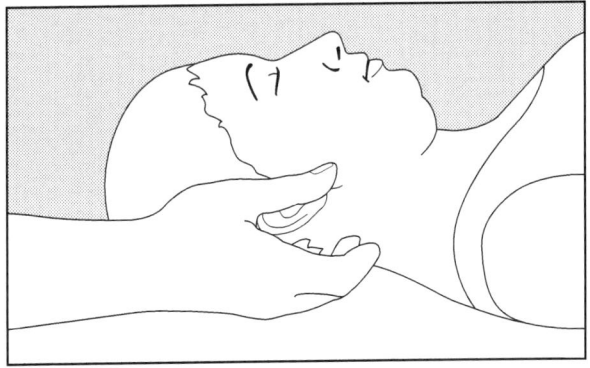

For example:

Step 1 Just as when working with your client prone, sit for a while with your fingers at the base of their skull. See if you can identify any differences between the left and right sides of the occipital bone, where trapezius inserts. Is one side more tender than the other? Move your fingertips off the bone and onto soft tissue, right at the base of the skull, the topmost part of the neck. How do the tissues feel? Experiment with the placement of your fingers and identify which is most comfortable for you when you remain in the same position for a few moments. Where do you need to rest your elbows in order to be comfortable? Does it make a difference how high or how low you position your treatment couch? Do you feel more comfortable sitting, kneeling, or squatting?

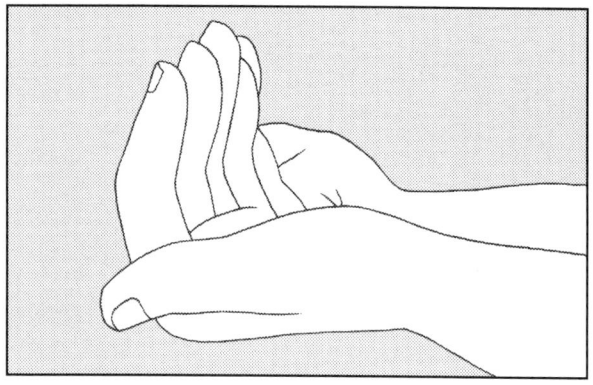

Step 2 Once you are comfortable, flex your metacarpophalangeal joints as shown here, taking the weight of the client's head onto your fingers, and let the head gently roll from side to side. Don't force any movements, instead, simply allow the client's head to move onto or off your fingertips. Does the head roll easily both to the left

and to the right, or does it get 'stuck' anywhere?
How does this gentle palpation-with-rocking feel
for your client? How does your own body feel
when you provide treatment in this position? Are
you comfortable or do you start to get backache?
It's important to safeguard your posture and you
may find that it takes a while to find that position
which is comfortable for both your back and for
your hands.

**Summary of questions to ask when treating
suboccipital muscles in the supine position**
- Do both left and right suboccipitals feel the same?
- If they feel different to you, in what way do they feel
  different? Is there an increase/decrease in tone on
  one side?
- Does the client report one side as being more
  tender than the other?
- Where do you need to rest your elbows, on or off
  the couch?
- Do you feel more comfortable sitting, kneeling or
  squatting?
- Does it make a difference if you raise/lower your
  treatment couch?

Side lying position

Another way to treat the suboccipital area is with your client in the side lying position. Here you can gently run your thumb from the base of the neck towards the occiput, dragging the skin gently in a cephalic direction and stopping when you reach the occipital bone. This is useful as it enables you to really focus on the suboccipital muscles on one side of the neck.

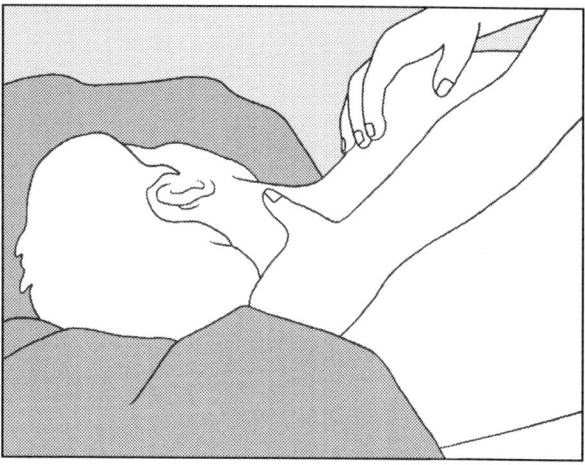

Experimenting with (or without) a pillow means you can practice this gentle stripping motion with the tissues of the posterior neck shortened (usually with a pillow) or lengthened and under a little tension (usually without a pillow).

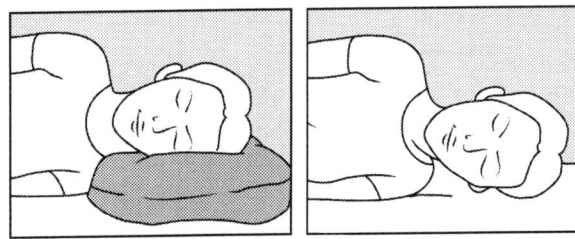

The advantage of not using a pillow, is that you can experiment with varying degrees of head flexion/extension, asking your client to perform a nodding motion.

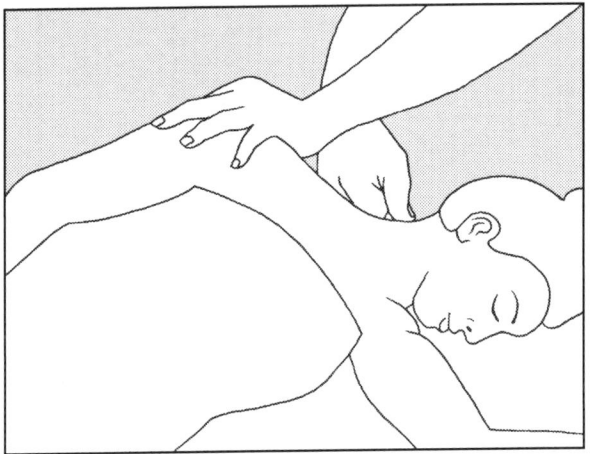

You can also practice changing the position of the client's arm. How does changing the position of the client's arm affect both you and your client?

Passively abducting the arm shortens the tissues spanning the arm and shoulder and with them slackened you can palpate to deeper structures. Alternatively, with the arm resting against the client's body, the tissues on the lateral side of the neck are tensioned, especially if you apply a little depression to the shoulder. Notice what happens when your client gently nods their head in this side lying position as you palpate the scalenes on one side of their neck. Sometimes you can facilitate relief simply by applying fingertip pressure as the client performs this rhythmic nodding movement.

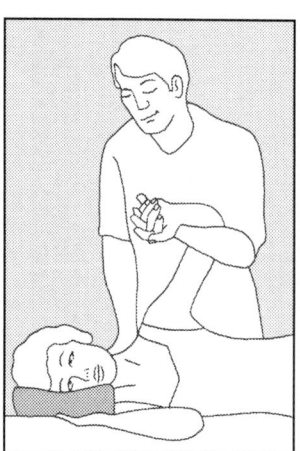

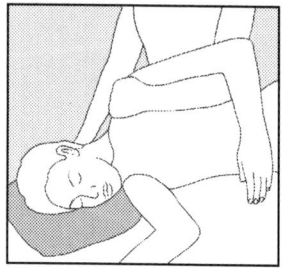

Seated

With your client seated, you can allow their head to fall gently back onto your thumbs and can thus apply gentle pressure to one side of the occipital

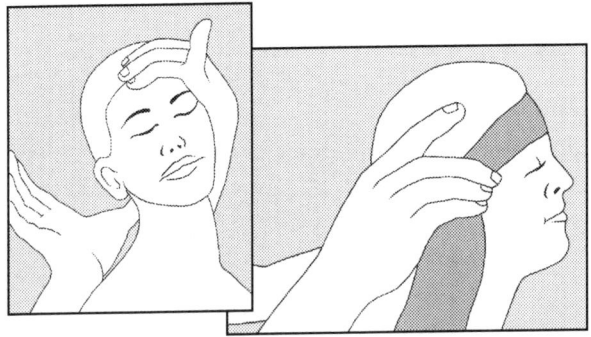

region at a time with relative ease to yourself. You will find that you need to support the client's forehead as shown. Whilst we need to guard against injury to our thumbs as therapists, this technique does not require deep pressure nor does it require you to rotate your thumb. Simply allow the suboccipital tissues to rest gently on your thumb for about 5-10 seconds before moving your thumb to a new position.

Ohashi (1977) suggests using a headband to help as you press your thumbs gently into the soft tissues of the occipital region. This area can be sore for many clients, so avoid holding any point for too long and avoid overworking the area in general.

Ohashi, W., 1977. Do-It-Yourself Shiatsu, London: Unwin Paperbacks

TIP 14 UNDERSTANDING LEVATOR SCAPULAE

Levator scapulae is an interesting muscle. It can be felt as a strap-like band running up the back of the neck on either side, deep to trapezius. Originating on the transverse processes of the upper three or four cervical vertebrae and inserting into the superior angle of the scapulae, when it is 'tight' it is palpable as a twangy band, about 2cm in width. Often, palpation and compression of this muscle elicits feelings of tenderness and relief simultaneously. As a result, it is tempting to massage this area deeply in an attempt to help stretch the muscle and not least because clients enjoy the sensation of relief such deep massage brings about. However, if we stop for a moment to consider the anatomy and function of levator scapulae it becomes

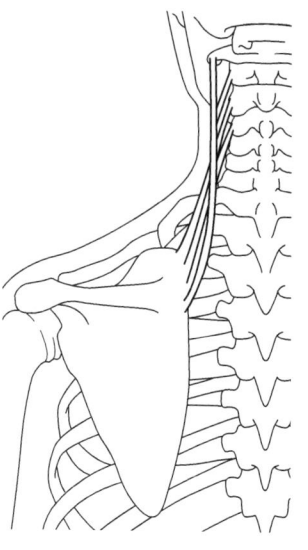

obvious that our attempts to lengthen this muscle
may not be advantageous.

Levator scapulae is very much like the reigns of a horse, and it often works to reign-in the head, helping to reposition the head over the thorax where it belongs, and where tension on supportive tissues is lessened. Often, when a client presents with a forward-head posture, craning their head as if hurrying, levator scapulae is forced to adopt a lengthened position. Tension in the muscle increases as it works *isometrically* to maintain head position, *eccentrically* as the head falls forward, and *concentrically* in an attempt to bring the head back over the body. It is not suprising that people with a forward head posture often complain of neck pain.

Whilst deep tissue massage and stretching are enjoyable to receive, and certainly help in reducing muscular tension, one of the long-term goals for clients with forward head posture is to help them to correct this posture and to shorten levator scapulae. For ideas on how clients can help to do this for themselves, please see *Neck Aftercare Tips, Tip 7, Neck Retractions* (pp.258-262).

TIP 15 ADDRESSING TRIGGER POINTS IN LEVATOR SCAPULAE

A useful technique for addressing pain and decreasing muscle tension in the neck is to palpate levator scapulae for trigger points and to try to reduce these. Sometimes this is achieved to great satisfaction if you position your client on their side and apply gentle pressure at a 90 degree angle onto the trigger point.

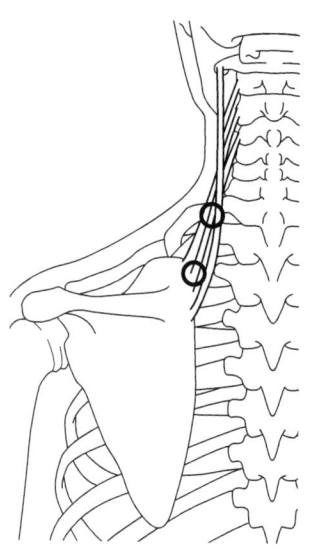

Trigger points in levator scapulae may also be addressed with your client prone or seated and it is worth experimenting with each to see which position works best for you.

Step 1 With your client in the chosen treatment position, start by warming up the area.

Step 2 Using light strokes to begin, cover the area slowly, and consistently, using your fingertips to search for trigger spots. If, after stroking the whole region you have not located any trigger points, repeat the process with slightly firmer strokes, palpating into a deeper layer of tissue. Remember to work *slowly*. Triggers will be discovered as palpable, tender points that often run in bands. They are often located close to where levator scapulae inserts onto the superior angle of the scapula.

Step 3 If you find a trigger point, rest your thumb or finger gently on the point and wait. Your client may feel some tenderness but should be able to tolerate your pressure without experiencing any pain. Within about 60 seconds you should feel a reduction in tension in this localized point and your client should report a decrease in tenderness. Soothe the area with massage before seeking out and treating another spot in the same manner.

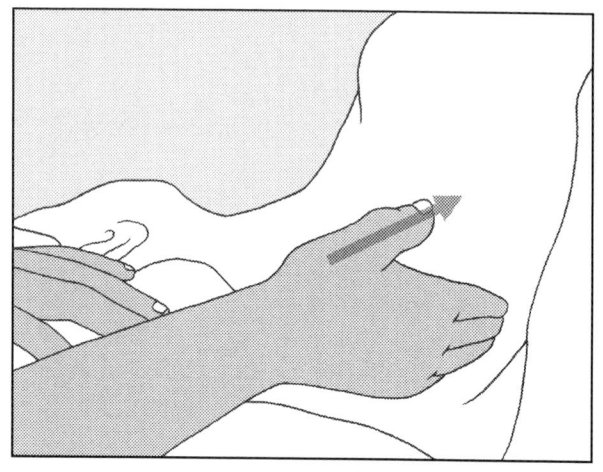

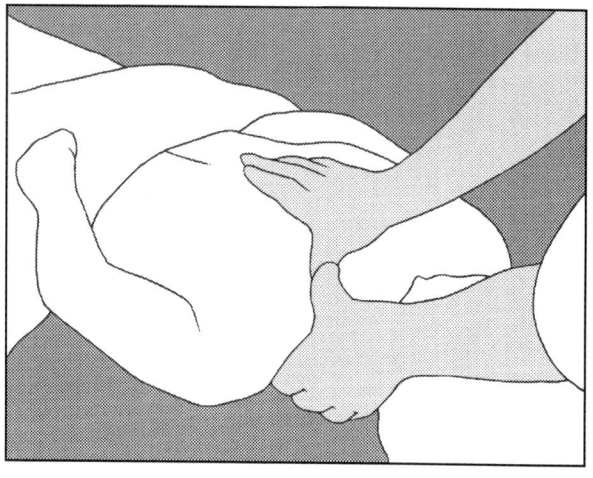

Tip It sometimes helps to encourage the client to imagine the tenderness simply melting away. Sometimes, with a verbal prompt such as this, both you and the client perceive this decrease in tone in the muscle.

Question: How long should I hold the trigger point for?

Hold the point until there is a decrease in tenderness. Usually this occurs within about 10-12 seconds but varies between individuals. If the trigger point is chronic it may take longer to 'release' but this is not always the case. Sometimes, the relief the client experiences simply from the pressure of gentle palpation at that particular point is so great that the decrease in muscle tone is apparent within seconds. At other times, you may find that you are holding a point for around 60 seconds and that any decrease in tone is very minor. The trick is not to try and force the release of a point. Again, working to the less-is-more principle, several attempts using light touch, can be more effective than trying to physically *push* a point away with brute force!

Many people find that a gentle neck stretch following the release of trigger points helps to 'reset' the muscle to its original length. This could be an active stretch or a passive stretch. Alternatively, simply taking the head through some of the cervical ranges of movement can be a nice way to finish a trigger point session.

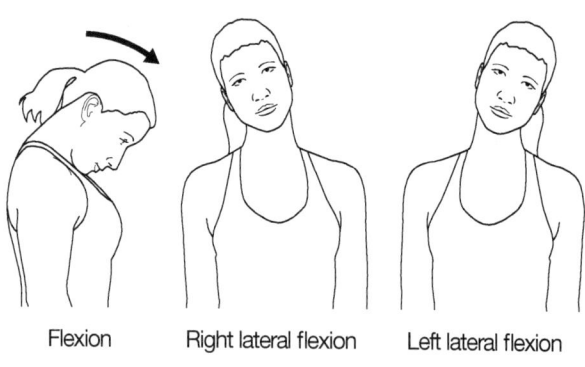

Flexion   Right lateral flexion   Left lateral flexion

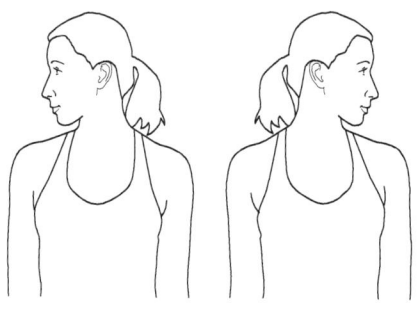

Right rotation   Left rotation

TIP 16 POSITIONAL RELEASE FOR LEVATOR SCAPULAE

If you discover tender spots in levator scapulae, one way to address these is to use a technique known as Positional Release or Strain-Counterstrain which was developed by a doctor of osteopathy, Lawrence Jones, and which involves repositioning your client so that their discomfort feels eased. You first need to identify the tender spot and then to passively slacken the soft tissues associated with this spot. In the case of levator scapulae, this means taking the client's head and neck into gentle lateral flexion on the side of the tenderness. With the neck laterally flexed and the shoulder passively elevated the fibers of levator scapulae are in a shortened position. There are a variety of ways to do this and it is likely that you will need to use a different treatment position for different clients. Once in the treatment position—seated, supine or side lying—you need to experiment to find the position in which your client feels *most* ease from their discomfort.

You can try this technique for yourself by following these very basic steps:

Step 1 With your client seated, find a comfortable position in which to passively elevate the scapula. This could be with your client seated next to a couch, their arm supported on the couch, or they could rest their arm over your thigh if you felt that that was appropriate for them. In this position, palpate for tender spots in levator scapulae. Rest your finger on a spot when you find one. If you are able to identify more than one spot, running in a band, choose the point in the middle.

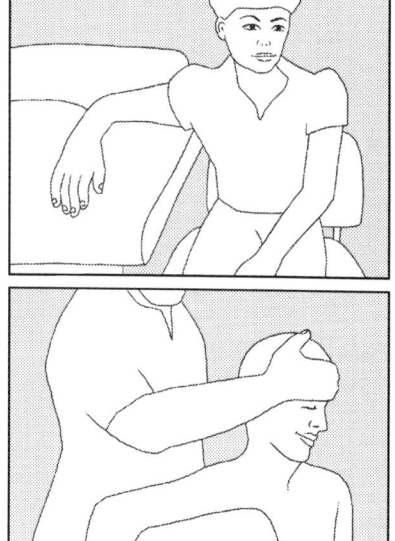

Step 2 Find the position of ease. Help place 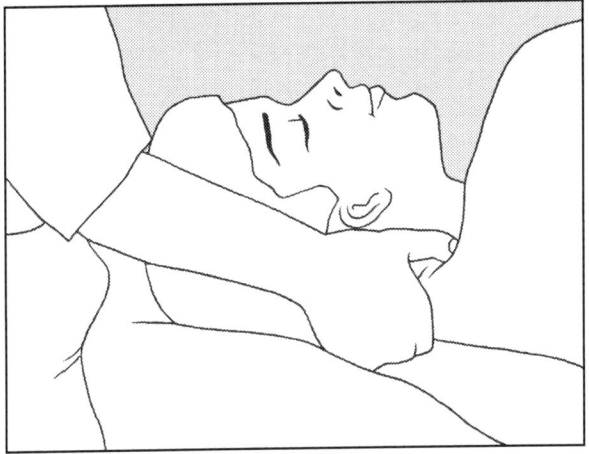levator scapulae into a passively shortened position by easing the client's head into lateral flexion, or extension, or rotation, or a combination of these movements. The client should report a 70% reduction in discomfort in the tender spot you are palpating once in the position of ease.

You may find this is easier to facilitate with the client in the side lying position which has the advantage of prompting greater relaxation and a reduction in muscle tone whereas when a client is

seated, the muscles of neck extension are active in order to support the weight of the head.

Step 3 Hold this position for 90 seconds while continuing to palpate the tender spot, and then gently return the client's head to the neutral position. In neutral, recheck the tender spot. There should be less discomfort on palpation.

Question: Are the tender spots that respond to *strain-counterstrain* the same as trigger points?

No. They are localized like trigger points, about 1cm in diameter, and represent either neuromuscular or musculoskeletal dysfunction but they do not respond to techniques such as Soft Tissue Release (described in the next tip) or to spray-and-stretch techniques. Nor do they respond to injections the way trigger points do.

For an interesting discussion on this topic, see Fallon, S. and Walsh, M., *Positional Release Technique, A valid technique for use by physical therapy practitioners?* IPTAS Conference (2012).

TIP 17 SOFT TISSUE RELEASE TO TRAPEZIUS/LEVATOR SCAPULAE

Another way to help decrease tone and stretch soft tissues in the posterior neck region is to use Soft Tissue Release (STR). This pin-and-stretch technique is helpful for alleviating the discomfort of trigger points. It is a relatively safe form of neck stretching because when STR is applied to the neck, it is the client who is in charge of how far they choose to stretch, not the therapist.

This tip explains how to apply STR to both trapezius and levator scapulae. In practice, these two muscles cannot be separated anatomically for the purposes of treatment, due to their fascial connections. Yet like other techniques (such as stretches and positional release technique), it is possible to place the focus of the technique more on one muscle than the other, bearing in mind that both will be affected, one to a lesser degree and one to a greater degree.

204 Focusing STR to trapezius

Step 1 Massage the upper back and neck to warm and soothe the tissues.

Step 2 Apply gentle pressure to the belly of the upper fibers of trapezius, avoiding bony points such as the clavicle and acromion process.

You can apply pressure using your thumb, finger, reinforced fingers, or, with caution, your elbow. In the illustration below, the therapist is using her forearm, attempting to gently compress the tissues, forming a 'lock'. She is standing behind the client using her right arm, but she could have chosen to stand to the side of the client and use her left arm.

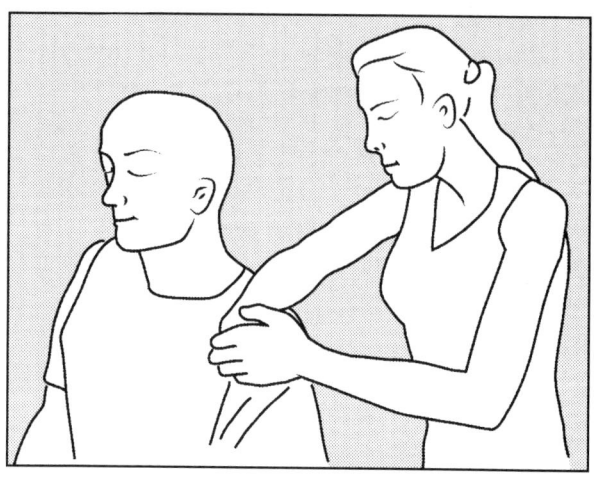

Step 3 While maintaining gentle pressure, ask your client to slowly take their head away from you. They should experience a stretch to the soft tissues to the side of their neck. Hold the position for about 10 seconds then release your lock and ask your client to return their head to neutral. Repeat two more times on this spot, or choose a different spot on which to work.

STR should be comfortable and pain free. There is sometimes slight tenderness but this should be tolerable. If the client experiences pain you should stop. Also, be cautious in using this technique on clients who have had problems such as lumbar herniations. Forces even from gentle compression of trapezius (or levator scapulae) are transmitted to the spine and could aggravate a pre-existing spinal condition.

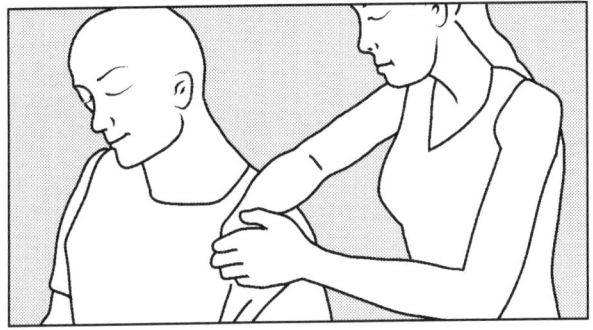

Focusing STR to levator scapulae

Here you will need to change the position of your lock so that you are more directly over this muscle. Also, the direction in which the client needs to stretch is different.

Step 1 As for the upper fibers of trapezius, locate an area of soft tissue and apply a gentle lock. Here the therapist has chosen to use her elbow to fix the tissues. Remember, using an elbow does not necessitate more force, it is simply a different 'tool' with which to apply the gentle 'lock'.

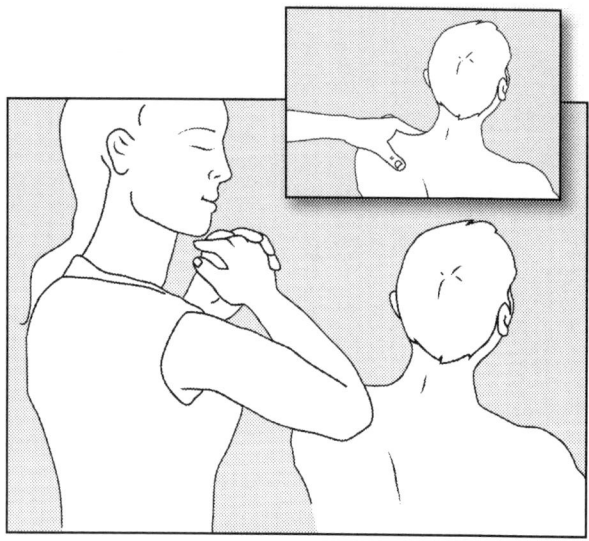

Step 2 While maintaining the lock, ask the client to rotate their head away from you about 45 degrees and then to look to the floor. They will experience a stretch of the posterolateral side of the neck. Soothe the area with general massage and then repeat STR on this same side, moving to a slightly different spot, or apply the stretch to the opposite side of the neck. Experiment with placing your lock in different positions on the neck and get feedback as to which head and neck movement the client needs to perform in order to experience the best sense of stretch and release.

Question: What if my client experiences referred sensations?

This technique should feel comfortable to receive and the client should experience a sense of relief following it. However, it is common for clients to report referred symptoms in other parts of their body such as the head, face, arm and chest. This is normal when there are trigger points present and your pressure is directly over a trigger point. The technique should never cause pain and if your client reports pain you should stop.

For more information on this technique, see Johnson, J., *Soft Tissue Release,* 2009. Champaign, IL: Human Kinetics

TIP 18 TREATING SCALENES

In *The Trigger Point Therapy Workbook* (2004, Oakland, CA, New Harbinger), author Clair Davies describes how trigger points located within the scalene muscles can refer pain to other parts of the body such as the arm, forearm, thumb, upper chest and scapula. To alleviate such discomfort, apply soft tissue release, using steps like those described here.

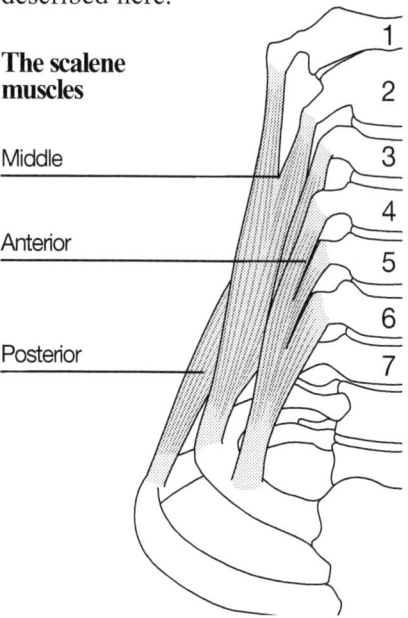

The scalene muscles

Middle

Anterior

Posterior

1
2
3
4
5
6
7

Step 1 Remind yourself about the anatomy of
scalenes and observe your client to see whether the
scalenes on one
side of the neck
are more
prominent at
rest. Following
the steps in
Part 1, Tip 14
(pp.70-71),
locate scalenes
on your subject.

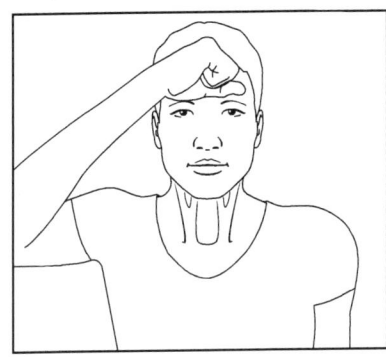

Step 2 Once you are
sure you have located a
scalene, use the pads of
your fingers to apply
gentle pressure to the
muscle superior to the
clavicle.

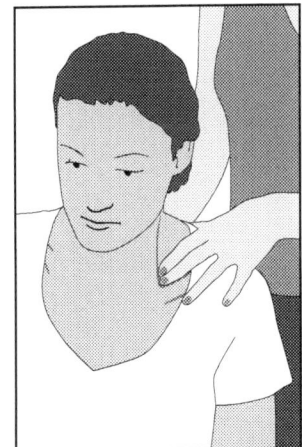

Step 3 Maintaining this gentle pressure, ask your client to turn their head away from your finger. Your subject should experience a mild stretch on the anterolateral side of their neck as they do this, releasing tension here. After a few seconds ask them to return their head to the start position (neutral) and repeat once more.

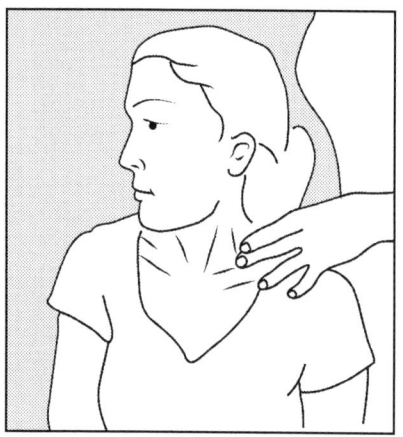

Palpate the scalenes on the opposite side of the neck. How does the tension in this side compare with the tension in the muscles you have just treated, is it increased or decreased? Apply soft tissue release to the opposite side of the neck. Check whether the application of this technique has increased the range of movement in your client's neck and/or decreased their discomfort.

TIP 19 TREATING SCM

Sternocleidomastoid (SCM) may become
hypertonic in clients with poor posture or
following whiplash injuries. It may be strained
during sporting activities and activities such as
overhead weightlifting. As it becomes active
during deep inspiration, when lung volume reaches
about 75%, and when a sudden intake of breath is
required, it can sometimes be seen in singers and
public speakers and is an important muscle of
respiration for people engaged
in heavy, physical activity.
Many clients do not realize
they have tension in their
sternocleidomastoid muscle
until they receive gentle
palpation and massage.

Although some therapists
choose to massage the length of
this muscle, it is wise to work
with sensitivity and caution
due to the proximity
of important
structures on the
anterior of the neck.

212 One way to treat sternocleidomastoid is to massage the area and then to apply a gentle stretch, placing one hand on the sternum, and applying slight traction with the other, at the side of the head. You can modify this stretch by gently rotating the head to one side and repositioning your hands.

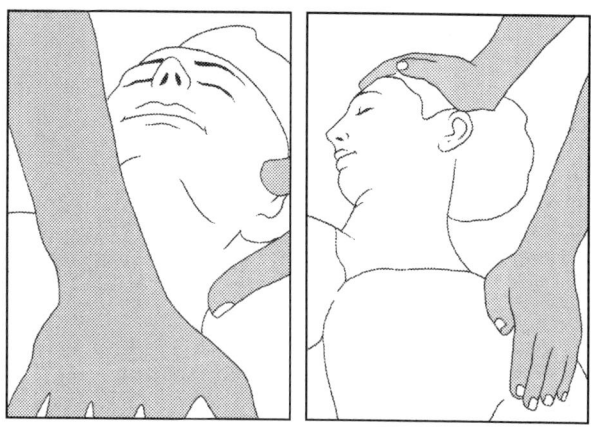

Tip Pressure on the belly of the muscle can stimulate a cough reflex and can make some clients feel uncomfortable, especially if both left and right sides of the neck were massaged at the same time. For this reason it is often more effective to restrict your treatment to gentle circling of the origins (sternum and clavicle) and insertion (mastoid process) of the muscle.

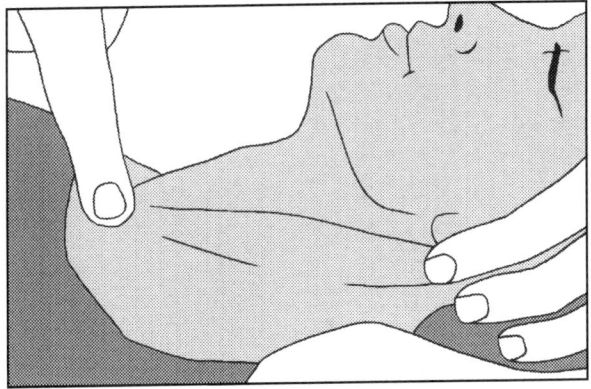For an interesting article on the activity patterns of sternocleidomastoid and latissimus dorsi in classical singers see Watson *et al* (2012). Also, Min *et al* (2010) provide a case study of a subject with auricular pain that was discovered to be derived from trigger points in sternocleidomastoid.

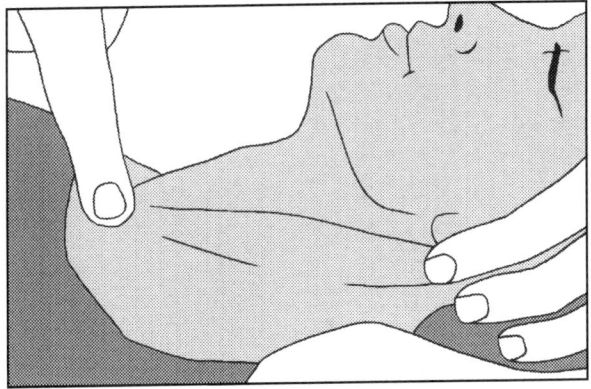

Watson, A.H.D., William, C., and James, B.V., 2012. Activity Patterns in Latissimus Dorsi and Sternocleidomastoid in Classical Singers. *Journal of Voice,* 2012 May; 26(3): e95–e105.

Min, S.H., Chang, S-H., Jeon, S.K., Yoon S.Z., Park J-Y., and Shin H.W., 2010. Posterior auricular pain caused by the trigger points in the sternocleidomastoid muscle aggravated by psychological factors - a case report. *Korean Journal of Anaesthesiology,* 2010 December; 59(Suppl): S229–S232.

TIP 20 MET TO THE NECK

Muscle Energy Technique (MET) is a form of stretching and strengthening. It has many applications and many variations and is useful when treating people with neck conditions. Included here are descriptions of two ways (bilateral and unilateral) in which you can use MET to help stretch muscles of the neck, specifically the muscles responsible for shoulder elevation and lateral flexion of the neck. Note that whilst the protocol described here uses a 10 second contraction and 10% of the client's force, this is only one method of applying MET, and one of the simplest. There are many variations of the technique and you are likely to come across therapists who use MET slightly differently. If you are new to this technique, try it and be prepared to modify it to suit your needs and those of your clients.

As MET requires the client to perform an isometric contraction, it should only be used on clients for whom it is safe. An example of a client for whom it may not be safe would be someone with unmedicated high blood pressure, as an increase in muscle tone increases blood pressure.

Supine, bilaterally

Use this method of application if your client is comfortable having both of their shoulders depressed at the same time.

Step 1 With your client comfortably positioned in the supine position, gently depress their shoulders, applying pressure caudally.

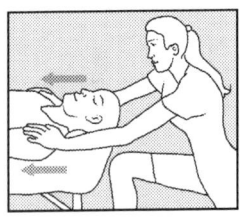

Step 2 Ask your client to shrug their shoulders, using about 10% of their force. Do not allow their shoulders to elevate. However, be wary of pushing their shoulders down. *You* are resisting the force provided by the client, the client should not be trying to resist you.

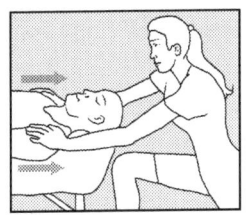

Step 3 After about 10 seconds, ask your client to relax, and then slowly depress their shoulders a little more. Hold them in this new, depressed position. Repeat once more if your client is willing.

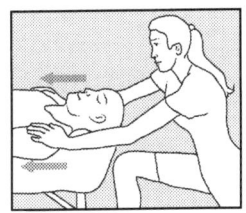

Tip: Instead of depressing the shoulders a second time, once your client has stopped shrugging, ask them to remain in the same position but to try and reach their hands toward their toes, depressing their own shoulders. This engages the lower fibers of trapezius as well as other muscles and can be helpful in decreasing tone in the upper fibers of this muscle.

The advantage of this method is that it saves time (you can stretch both sides of the neck at once) and it can be useful when stretching the neck muscles of clients who are hypermobile and for whom the supine unilateral stretch is not appropriate. The disadvantage is that it cannot be used with clients who have an acute shoulder injury such as supraspinatus tendinosus, acromioclavicular joint injuries, injury to the lateral third of the clavicle or subdeltoid bursitis, as it does require some pressure, albeit gentle, to be applied to the head of the humerus.

Supine, unilaterally
Use this method of application if your client has a shoulder problem and you think bilateral MET may aggravate this. Or, simply use it as an alternative to depressing the shoulders bilaterally.

Step 1 With your client comfortably positioned in the supine position, place one hand on their shoulder and another on the side of their 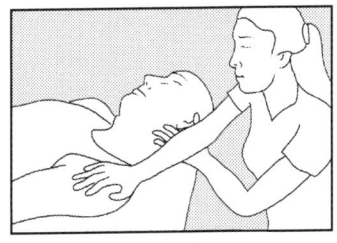 face. Gently apply pressure, taking their head into lateral flexion.

Step 2 Keeping your hands here, the head and shoulder fixed, ask your client to try to bring their head back to a neutral position, while 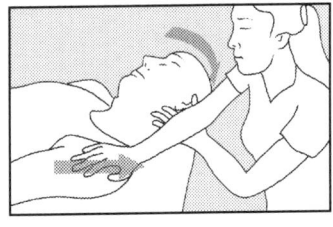 shrugging their shoulder, using about 10% of their force. You can see that this engages the lateral flexors of the neck. Again, be wary of pushing your client's head and shoulder apart: *You* should be resisting the force provided by your client, your client should not be trying to resist you.

Step 3 After about 10 seconds, ask your client to relax, and then slowly take the neck a little more into lateral flexion.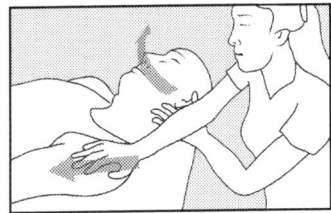

Hold the head in this new position, encouraging your client to breath normally and relax. If a client has a very stiff neck, with a decreased range of lateral flexion, you may wish to perform this again on the same side. However, the neck does not require a great deal of gross lateral flexion so it is sometimes better to err on the side of caution and apply other techniques to help loosen stiffness and increase range of movement, than to attempt to stretch the neck again using MET. Repeat on the other side of the neck.

The advantage of this method is that it can be used to help stretch the neck of a client who cannot receive MET bilaterally. The disadvantages are that it can be too severe for some clients and care must be taken not to overstretch the tissues. For this reason it is not appropriate for clients who are hypermobile, who already have a good range of movement into lateral flexion of their neck. Another disadvantage is that when the neck is taken into lateral flexion, muscles are shortened on one side of the neck and they risk cramping.

TIP 21 TAPING THE NECK

Neck Treatment Tips ends with a tip about tape. It is a tip designed to raise questions and to stimulate your thinking!

The use of tape to help improve muscle function is not new but is becoming increasingly popular due to new versions of tape that are now available to therapists. If you intend to use tape with the intention of helping a client to improve function or to decrease pain in their neck, you should consider undertaking special training. However, you should also bear in mind that results for the use of tape are mixed. Whilst certain types of tape are valuable in restricting movement, there is less evidence for the use of tape to decrease pain and to enhance movement. For this reason, it is difficult to describe a specific protocol for the use of tape when treating clients with neck conditions.

The starting point when considering the use of tape as a therapeutic modality should be to ask yourself for what purpose is it being used? What are your therapeutic goals?

Examples of therapeutic goals are:

> to decrease pain
> to decrease discomfort
> to decrease stiffness
> to decrease muscle tone
> to increase muscle tone
> to improve range of movement
> to improve function (as in activities of daily living or sporting function)
> to help correct postural imbalance

Ask yourself next whether there are other interventions that would be as good as, or better than the application of tape.

A common condition you may already have come across is that of a forward head posture, with clients complaining of pain and soreness in their neck and shoulders as a result of muscle imbalance. It seems reasonable to assume that tape could be used to help the client maintain a better head and neck posture if the tape were applied in such a way as to temporarily correct posture and discourage the 'chin' poke position many people fall into. In this example, tape could be applied to the upper trapezius in such a manner that when the client's posture falters, and they start craning forward, the tape is tensioned and they are alerted to correct their posture. However, it needs to be remembered that tape is thought to stimulate mechanoreceptors and in doing so is likely to increase tone in muscles. Is this what you would want to achieve in the upper fibers of trapezius in a client with poor posture?

Some tape manufacturers claim that their tape can be used to decrease muscle tone if it is applied in a particular manner. If you wanted to decrease tone in the upper fibers of trapezius, for example, would using tape be your best treatment approach or could you use another treatment modality to achieve this goal?

Part 3 Neck Aftercare
Tips & Tricks

It can be a struggle sometimes, to know what to say to a client who is in pain with a recent neck injury, or who has been suffering with a neck problem for many months or years. Often clients want a 'quick fix' or they are fearful of re-injury and scared to move their neck at all. Sometimes a person is simply worn down by the constant discomfort of a chronic neck condition, or with having to cope with a neck condition that flares up unexpectedly.

The 11 *tips* in this final part of the book are all about the kinds of information you can give to your clients to help them to manage their neck conditions. This includes information you can provide to help explain their condition and how best to recover from neck problems, advice on safe stretches and simple exercises they can perform, as well as a few tricks you may not have come across. *Part 3* begins with tips about how we can help educate, advise and reassure clients by throwing light on neck care facts which you, as a therapist, may take for granted, but about which clients may not be aware.

As therapists it is probable that we are more informed about the body than most of our clients, and an important part of our role is to help educate people as to how they can prevent, manage, and resolve their symptoms. Of course, there are many clients with a high level of understanding about anatomy and physiology, and about injury and rehabilitation, especially if they are keen on being able to take part in a regular physical activity and want to lessen their chances of injury. However, even when a client is a regular exerciser and is fairly well-informed, this does not mean that they have the same knowledge and appreciation about their bodies as we do as therapists. It is common for clients to use the internet to seek solutions to their neck problems. The internet is not only a fantastic source for sharing knowledge, it also contains much mis-information. We have an ideal opportunity to help clients care for their necks and manage their neck complaints in a safe and appropriate way.

TIP 1 PLAYING SHERLOCK

One of the reasons neck problems persist can be because a client continues to do something that aggravates their symptoms. Aggravating and easing factors are usually identified during the initial assessment and the information used to help identify the condition with which the client is suffering. The identification of aggravating factors is included here, as part of aftercare, because it often requires the client to take concerted action, outside of the therapy clinic, in order to determine what these aggravating factors are. Often a client can tell you immediately which movements, activities or conditions give rise to more discomfort, pain or a 'flare up' of their neck problem, but in some cases they cannot. Sometimes, an aggravating factor is an activity that is so commonplace that the client fails to recognize it as an aggravating factor at all. The longer a person has been doing an activity, and the more commonplace it is for them, the less likely they are to consider it an aggravating factor. This is how as therapists, we can help by asking open-ended questions that may prompt awareness.

Further, the aggravating factor does not necessarily need to involve movement. Where a task involves a person keeping their neck in a static position for a long period of time, this too can be problematic. Examples of when the head and neck are held static or almost static are reading, using a microscope, bird watching, concentrating on close-work hobbies such as needlecraft, sitting at a desk using a laptop or computer and watching television.

Question: What if my client cannot identify any aggravating factors?

A useful tip here is to suggest that your client keeps an activity diary for 7 days, for a period of time that represents their normal routine. When the client returns for another appointment with you, ask them what it was they were doing when their symptom came on, and try to get as specific as possible. Were they moving or staying still? If they were moving, what were they doing? Can they remember which movement they did, did it involve their neck only or did it involve their arms or shoulders too? Were they lifting or carrying anything, for example? Was it a whole body activity, were they engaged in sport or exercise? If they told you, for example, that it came on when they were swimming, what stroke were they doing? A common example of a stroke that aggravates neck pain in some people is when the client does breaststroke while keeping their head above the water, their neck in extension. If the activity involved moving only their head, what did they do – ask them in layperson's terms whether they looked down (flexion), up to the ceiling (extension), over one shoulder (rotation), etc. Was it a combination of movements? If the client was in a static position when the symptom came on, what were they doing? Where they standing or sitting, crouching or lying? If they were lying, in which position, on their back, side or on their stomach? If the symptom came on when they were lying on their stomach with their head turned to the right, for example, does the symptom also come on when they rest prone with their head to the left? If they were sitting, what were they doing? Were they reading? Watching television? Did they fall asleep? If they fell asleep and woke up with neck pain, where was their head and neck when they woke up, had it dropped forward or to one side?

Where a symptom develops from a static posture you will need to help the client identify whether it is the posture itself that aggravates the symptom or whether the symptom is duration-dependent. For example, if a person's pain comes on when they remain static in order to read, for how long can they read (remain in this posture) before the symptom develops?

Once you have specific information concerning aggravating factors you are a short step away from providing the client with preventative advice.

Question: Do clients really need help identifying aggravating factors?

It may seem obvious that if a symptom develops after retaining a static posture for 40 minutes, for example, the solution is simply to avoid this position for more than say, 30 minutes. Yet we all fall victim to these kinds of habits and having someone point out that we are sitting too long, for example, is a good thing. You have probably come across plenty of clients who will tell you, "Yeah, I know, you're right, it's just that when I'm into it I can't seem to stop," or, "I forgot the time". Maybe a solution would be to print a line of copy in books which says, "Stop, you have read 100 pages, do you need to take a break?" (By the way, if you are reading these *Neck Tips* cover-to-cover, stop, you have read 227 pages.)

Useful exploratory questions to help identify aggravating factors

Use these questions to prompt your own thinking and to help you when questioning clients in order to try and identify aggravating factors which you can then eliminate or reduce. These are by no means exhaustive, and are in no particular order, but will hopefully provide a jumping off point for further investigation.

When you noticed your symptom:

Where you moving or staying still?

If you were moving, what were you doing?

Can you remember which movement you did, did it involve your neck only or did it involve you arms or shoulders too?

Were you lifting or carrying anything?

Were you shrugging your shoulders?

Where were your arms, were they hanging loose by your sides, supported on a chair or in some other position?

Did you notice your symptom following a whole body activity such as sport or exercise? If so, what were you doing and which part of the activity aggravated the symptom? For example, if you were swimming, what stroke were you doing?

If you moved only your head before the symptom came on, what did you do – did you look down (flexion), up to the ceiling (extension), over one shoulder (rotation) or was it some other movement? Can you show me what you did?

If you were in a static position when the symptom came on, what were you doing? Where you standing or sitting, crouching or lying?

If you were lying, in which position, on your back, side or stomach? In which position was your head and neck? Can you show me?

If you were sitting, what were you doing? How were you sitting, upright, or slumped, on a chair or on a sofa, at work, the cinema, in a cafe or at home? Can you show me how you were sitting?

Were you reading, watching television or doing a craft activity? Can you show me the position you were in when doing this activity?

Did you fall asleep sitting? Where was your head and neck when you woke up, had it dropped forward or to one side?

For how long can you remain in this static posture before the symptom develops?

Question: Why do we need to bother being so <u>specific</u> in trying to identify aggravating factors?

Firstly, aggravating factors help us as clinicians to determine the condition we are dealing with, and secondly, once we know what aggravates a person's symptoms we can help them to find ways to eliminate or avoid these things.

Example of how getting specific information can help identify aggravating factors

A client comes to you with a recurring neck problem and tells you they cannot identify anything that makes it worse. As part of your home care advice you suggest that they keep a 7-day diary and when they return a week later they tell you that they still cannot identify what's aggravating their pain, only that, "It came on when I went to see my neighbor". You ask what they were doing and they reply, "I wasn't doing anything different. It was a normal day." Your task is to be the Sherlock Holmes of therapists, to discover what was different that particular day, that particular occasion. Has visiting their neighbor ever triggered this symptom before? What are they doing when they visit, is the trigger to do with how they sit or stand at a neighbor's house? You ask the client to tell you exactly what they did,

("Just the usual. We had coffee.") so you ask, "Was
anything different that day at all?" What would
you think if they then said, "Nothing. Only I didn't
have my scarf that day"?

"Do you usually wear a scarf?", you ask. They tell
you that they always wear a scarf and when you
ask, "Why?" they say, "I don't know, I just feel
better with it on."

"So what happened when you visited your
neighbor that day you didn't have a scarf on?"

"Nothing, but my neck started hurting."

"What were you doing?"

"Drinking coffee."

Then the client remembers, "It was cold".

So now you are faced with an opportunity: was the
symptom brought on by holding a particular
posture to drink coffee, retaining this posture for a
long period of time, sitting to drink coffee in a
cold environment, or was it something altogether
different that also happened while at the neighbor's
house that triggered the neck pain. Later the client
says, "Come to think of it, I think the cold does
make it worse." You ask them to explain. "When I
go to the cinema I can't sit in an aisle seat because
if there's a draft my neck hurts." Then they
remember that when they sat in a restaurant one
time under some air conditioning vent they had
neck pain the following day.

You can see that from the information generated in this particular example, you are starting to build up a picture of causal factors and might surmise that the client has a neck condition aggravated by cold temperatures. This kind of questioning and the responses the client gives help your client realize just how important it is for them to keep their neck warm.

Although identification of aggravating factors is part of your initial assessment, you can see now how encouraging a client to identify aggravating factors themself is key to successful intervention.

Identifying obsolete exercises

A client may be reluctant to consider that an exercise they have been doing regularly could be an aggravating factor, especially if it was an activity which they took up initially to help overcome a problem, and which seemed to help alleviate the problem at the time.

Example 1 A client may have once been advised to do neck 'rolls', circumducting their head which at the time alleviated their symptoms. Perhaps they were retaining a static posture for long periods of time and neck rolls were a way of alleviating tension in the muscles of the neck and shoulders?

Perhaps they had a stiff neck and a reduced range
of movement and so neck rolls were given as a
means of encouraging the client to move through,
and improve, all ranges. Three years later,
performing end of range neck rolls every hour
while sitting a their desk may not be appropriate.

Example 2 A client may have been told as a child
that doing headstands is good for core stability and
would help keep their neck strong. Years later,
trying to do headstands as part of a neck
strengthening regime following a whiplash
accident is probably not advisable.

Clients sometimes continue to perform exercises
prophylactically, believing these likely to prevent
their symptoms returning. Whilst some neck
exercises are useful to perform regularly, most are
prescribed to help manage a specific condition, at
a specific point in time in the course of a person's
recovery. Many clients stick to old regimes
believing these to be helpful when these may at
best be ineffective now, or at worst are aggravating
a condition. One of your tasks is to help identify
where a client is performing an exercise that has
long since become obsolete for the client's needs,
and to help educate them in this.

TIP 2 ACUTE VERSUS CHRONIC: BASIC ADVICE

Advice for clients with either acute or chronic neck pain

- Reassure your client that X-rays and MRI scans often reveal degenerative changes in the cervical vertebrae. It would be wrong to assume that a neck problem is due solely to these changes. Many people whose necks show signs of degeneration are problem free, experience no pain and no stiffness. Degenerative change is normal and happens to us all as we age.
- Reassure your client by telling them that the neck often makes a creaking sound known as 'crepitus'. This does not necessarily mean there is anything wrong.
- Reassure your client that there is much that can be done to help them, and many different interventions they can try. As a therapist, consider the main problem—is it pain, stiffness, impairment of function, etc.—and brainstorm all of the things you know are useful in addressing each of these.
- Ask your client to consider the general advice provided here as well as the advice on staying active.

Advice for a client with acute neck pain

- Most acute neck pain resolves at best within a few days, at worst within a few weeks.
- The sooner you return to normal daily activities the sooner you are likely to get better.
- The sooner you are able to move your neck, the sooner you are likely to get better.
- People who avoid moving their neck and avoid returning to their daily activities are at greater risk of suffering chronic neck pain and report coping less well with their pain.
- People who start moving and who try to return to normal are likely to recover quickly and to cope best with neck pain.
- Modify your activities to start with.
- When we damage the outside of our bodies we see evidence of damage—a wound, bruise, scab or scar. When we damage the insides of our body, we can't see the damage. The body needs time to heal on the inside just as on the outside, with blood vessels, muscles, tendons and ligaments, and in some cases, fractures repairing themselves, and nerve inflammations settling down. Pain often resolves before the healing process is complete so most of the time we simply need to be patient.
- Most causes of neck pain are not serious.

Advice for a client with chronic neck pain

- For clients who suffer isolated episodes of pain, try to discover if there is a trigger. Encourage your client to try and pinpoint what brought on their pain. If necessary, review *Part 3*, *Tip 1* to see if you can identify aggravating factors and remove or eliminate these.

- If the pain is due to an underlying condition such as degenerative changes in cervical vertebrae, remind your client that between episodes they often experience weeks or even months when they are pain-free or have much reduced levels of pain.

- If you feel it is appropriate, ask your client to consider pain medication as one way of managing if their pain is constant. Medication may not need to be taken all of the time but can be a useful way of helping clients to cope.

- For clients suffering chronic pain, suggest they consider trying to pace their activities, reducing the duration or intensity of what they do. For example, make several shopping trips, carrying lighter shopping each time.

- Suggest a client considers attending a pain management clinic. Techniques such as Cognitive Behavioural Therapy are an established means of helping people to manage long-term pain.

Unless a client has an acute and potentially dangerous neck condition, the general advice provided here is likely to be safe and helpful.

Recommendation	Rational
Relative rest	Resting for more than one or two days is not usually helpful for people with neck pain.
Stay physically active	There are tremendous benefits for people with neck pain in staying physically active. Consider all forms of exercise that are deemed safe for that particular person, such as walking, swimming, and stretching classes. Remaining physically active does not have to involve formal exercise classes or sport. Walking to and from work or to and from the cinema, or to the shops instead of taking a car or public transport constitutes physical activity. Could your client do a home DVD exercise program? Could they walk their own or a friend's dog? Try to think 'outside the box' and ask not what they can't do, but what your client *can* do. How could you work with a fitness professional to help them increase their levels of physical activity? How could they increase this themselves on a daily basis?
Maintain active range of movement (continues over)	Whilst some people feel safer if they minimize the extent to which they move their head, in the long term avoidance of all neck movements is not usually advisable as muscles atrophy with disuse and are therefore less able to support the head. Collars that keep the neck

Recommendation	Rational
(continued) Maintain active range of movement	immobile are therefore not helpful long term. Even small movements can help reduce discomfort and improve recovery times.
Avoid aggravating factors	Help your client to identify which movements and activities most aggravate their neck. Consider ways to avoid or minimize these. For example, if they remain stationary for long periods of time ask whether the task they are doing could be broken into smaller segments. Could they split up this activity throughout the day? Or, could they do some stretches or movements to overcome this static position.
Use heat or cold for pain relief	The application of heat and cold can be used for pain relief and which of them is used depends largely on the client's preferences. In acute situations cold is usually applied, and it has a general numbing effect on the body and thus decreases pain. However, applying cold to the neck region is not always pleasant and could give some clients a headache. For this reason it should be applied for a short duration only, for a few minutes if tolerable. Caution is needed to avoid using heat at too high a temperature or for too long a period. Heat is useful for decreasing muscle spasm, one of the contributing factors to pain. Performing neck ranges of movement or gentle neck stretches may be easier after the application of heat.

Recommendation	Rational
Avoid feeling cold	When we are cold we tend to shrug our shoulders and this increases the tone in neck muscles. It is therefore important to keep well wrapped up in cold weather and to identify risks such as when the client is in an air-conditioned environment. Some clients with neck pain are particularly susceptible to cold. What preventive measures do they use? Do they avoid certain environments? Carry a scarf? Carry a heat pack?
Encourage relaxation	Feeling stressed or angry increases muscle tone and is likely to aggravate some neck conditions. Finding ways to relax physically and emotionally is important in helping to manage neck conditions and help aid recovery. Consider asking your client to think constructively about how they could build rest and relaxation into their rehabilitation program, just as they might plan neck exercises.

TIP 3 GET CLIENTS MOVING

The message here is that unless a client has suffered an acute injury, or has neck pain resulting from a serious pathology such as a herniated cervical disk, cervical fracture or tumor, for example, movement and exercise is better for them than immobility.

THE ADVANTAGES OF ACTIVITY AND DISADVANTAGES OF INACTIVITY FOR PEOPLE WITH NECK PAIN	
Advantages of activity	**Disadvantages of inactivity**
Helps maintain and improve range of movement in the neck	Is likely to lead to a decreased range of movement in the neck
May help reduce feelings of stiffness	Is likely to increase feelings of stiffness
May help reduce pain	May increase pain
Helps elevate a person's mood	May contribute to feelings of depression

(continued) **Advantages of activity**	(continued) **Disadvantages of inactivity**
Helps maintain and improve muscle strength	Results in muscles weakening
Helps maintain and improve proprioception in the joints of cervical vertebrae and can help maintain and improve balance	Is likely to lead to a reduction in proprioception in joints of cervical vertebrae and a reduction in balance
Movement promotes blood flow to muscles, tendons and ligaments, aids lymph drainage and stimulates repair	Decreased blood flow to muscles, tendons and ligaments combined with reduced lymph drainage is likely to increase scar tissue and hinder repair
Can help a client feel that they are in control and making progress	Can lead to feelings of helplessness and lack of progress

Advice for clients on how to incorporate neck movement into their daily activities without aggravating an existing neck condition	
Sleeping	On waking, lie on your back and gently roll your head from one side to the other. Next, sit on the edge of the bed and take your neck through its range of movement—flexion, extension, rotation left and right and lateral flexion left and right, performing each movement one or two times. Neck and shoulder muscles are connected so perform one or two shoulder shrugs or shoulder rolls. Together these movements can help get the joints of your neck moving and help you feel a little looser before you start your day.
Driving	Holding your head, neck and shoulders stationary for long periods of time increases muscle tension and can aggravate certain neck conditions. Consider how to drive less—consider fewer journeys or journeys of shorter duration. Can you use other forms of transport or get a lift for all or some of your journey? If you have to drive, or have a particularly long journey planned, break up the journey as much as possible, stopping to rest. During these rests perform simple range of movement neck movements, stretches, and shoulder shrugs or shoulder rolls. Adjust your seat so that you are as comfortable as possible before your journey.
Commuting and traveling	It's important to keep your neck moving, avoiding a static posture for long periods of time. Range of movement exercises and shoulder shrugs can be performed surreptitiously if you are concerned about people watching you, on a station platform or while waiting at an airport. If you need to

(continued) Commuting and traveling	travel on a crowded bus, train or tram, sit if a seat is available so that you can avoid holding a bar or strap for support as elevation of the shoulder requires some neck and shoulder muscles to contract and shorten and in some cases this can lead to spasming of the muscle. This may be more likely to happen if you are prone to neck spasms. If you have to hold onto something by raising your arm, avoid using the arm on the side of your neck that spasms, or change arms where possible; practice depressing your shoulder blades a couple of times while you are holding on, contracting muscles opposite to those that are prone to spasm.
Watching TV	Avoid remaining stationary without moving your neck for periods of more than about 40 minutes. Use commercial breaks as a prompt to perform simple neck movements and shoulder shrugs. Avoid sitting for long periods with your head turned to one side, even slightly. Is your TV screen in front of you or do you need to turn to watch it? Having to look up, to a wall-mounted screen, or down, to a screen close to the floor, for long periods of time increases muscle tension and is likely to aggravate certain neck conditions. Where possible, have your furniture rearranged so that your TV screen is in front of you and the top of the screen is level with your eyes.
Working at a desk (continued over)	As with watching TV, avoid remaining stationary without moving your neck for periods of more than about 40 minutes. Don't wait to feel stiff and sore before moving. Move before that happens! Take regular micro breaks—30 seconds or so—and use these to perform simple neck movements and shoulder shrugs. Use a visual or auditory screen alert as a reminder for when its time to

(continued) Working at a desk	take a break. Check that any screen you are using is in front of you and that the top of the screen is level with your eyes. Where possible, vary the type of work you are doing so that you change the position of your neck. For example, swap between typing and writing and speaking on the telephone. If you know that your neck starts to ache or spasm when in the draft from air conditioning or a window, get into the habit of always carrying a lightweight scarf with you that you can use as and when needed. Shoulder and neck muscles are connected, and overreaching for things on your desk could aggravate your neck condition. Move things closer to you where possible.
Hobbies	If a hobby requires you to keep your neck stationary for long periods of time, such as reading, needlework, painting or fine model making, stop and take breaks every 40 minutes or so. Set a watch or phone alert to remind you when it's time to take a break during which you can move your neck and shoulders. Dog walkers report that sometimes a sharp tug on the leash can trigger their neck pain. Solutions are to swap the hand in which you hold the leash, or to use an extendable leash.
Daily activities and chores	Lifting and carrying can aggravate some neck conditions as the load is transmitted through the arms and shoulders to muscles spanning both the shoulder and neck. Minimize what you need to lift and to carry, carry items close to your body or not at all — use a wheelie case or buggy or backpack. When we carry a heavy bag on one shoulder we tend to shrug that shoulder and this can aggravate some neck conditions and lead to spasming of the

(continued) Daily activities and chores	muscles on that side. If you have to carry a bag, try changing hands and swap the shoulder on which you carry it. Avoid holding a phone on one side of the head for long periods of time as such use tends to cause us to laterally flex to that side and this too can lead to spasming of muscles on that side. Where possible, minimize using the phone in this way or change the way you use it—convert to speaker phone, headset or Skype for example. Certain daily activities can trigger spasm in neck muscles where the activity involves lifting a weight on one side, or raising one or both arms above the head. For example, holding a hair dryer to the head, reaching up to put crockery into a cupboard, reaching up to hang drapes, hanging washing on a line, reaching up to wash a window. In the acute stages, avoid these activities. Avoid or minimize time spent vacuuming or ironing, activities that involve repetitive movement of the arms combined with a fairly static neck posture.
Exercise and sports	Exercise and sports help people cope with pain, and help in the rehabilitation process. Impact and contact activities are potentially aggravating for people with neck conditions, so non-impact and non-contact are preferable. Sports and exercise do not have to be stopped, simply modified. Ways to modify these are to change the activity itself (e.g. from cycling to walking), to change the intensity of the activity (e.g., every other day rather than every day) or the duration of the activity (e.g., 20 minutes a day instead of 60 minutes a day). Some activities can be modified to reduce their impact, for example, instead of doing breaststroke when swimming, change to backstroke.

TIP 4 SIMPLE NECK STRETCHES

The most simple stretches you can give a client are active Range of Movement (ROM) stretches. Whilst ROM tests are used as part of cervical assessment, actively moving the neck through its normal ranges will constitute a stretch for some clients and they should practice these before attempting other stretches.

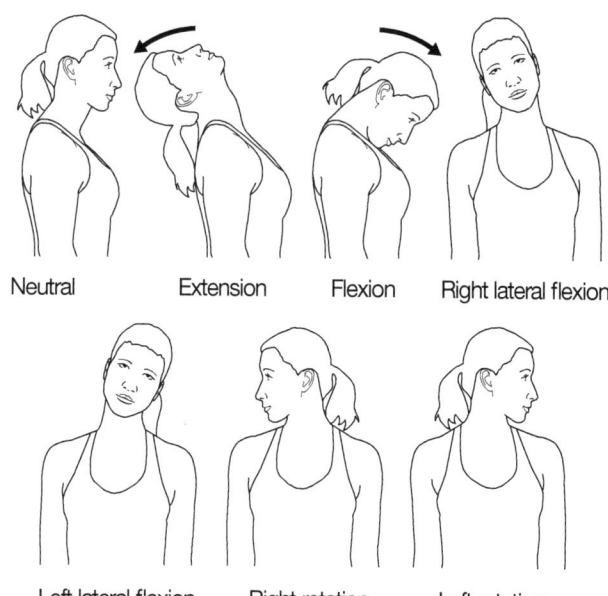

Neutral   Extension   Flexion   Right lateral flexion

Left lateral flexion   Right rotation   Left rotation

Follow this simple plan for increasing range of movement in the neck:

1. Encourage your client to perform the movements of flexion, extension, right rotation, left rotation, right lateral flexion and left lateral flexion, moving slowly, only as far into each range as they feel comfortable. Once the client is comfortable moving their neck, ask them to hold each position when they get to that point where they are starting to feel slight discomfort. Encourage them to repeat these movements throughout the day, following the maxim, *little and often*.

2. Once the client is confident in attempting the ROM movements, no matter how slight or how reduced in range, encourage them to increase the range slightly. Do this by suggesting that with each movement, as they approach the point at which they feel discomfort, they move gently one or two millimeters further into the range. This may be uncomfortable but should not hurt and if a client reports pain or dizziness then of course they should stop.

Ask your client to practice these ROM stretches regularly throughout the day, and over the coming week to take note of any improvements. Improvements might come in the form of:

- being able to move through a greater range
- being able to move through the same range with less pain
- being able to move through the same range with less hesitancy
- being able to move through the same range with less stiffness or less dizziness, etc.

Remember that it's important for the client to keep their shoulders still, not to twist at the waist or raise their shoulders to facilitate the movement.

It can be helpful to give a client a diary (example shown right) to complete which can act as a reminder and onto which they can note:

- any increases in range,
- any problems, or
- how many times they were able to perform a particular movement.

	Monday	Tuesday	Wednesday	Thursday	Friday	Saturday	Sunday

Alternative ways to increase cervical ROM
One way to increase active cervical rotation is for a client to lie on their back and to gently rotate their head to the left and to the right while it is supported by a bed or the floor.

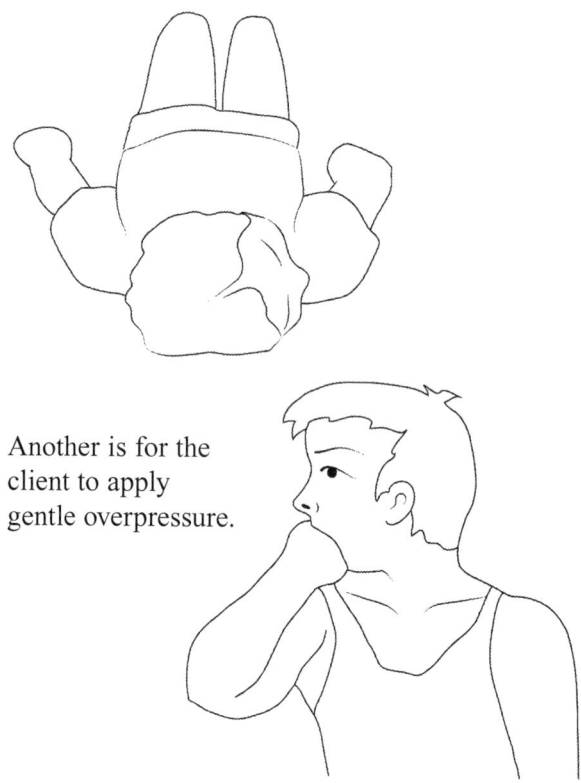

Another is for the client to apply gentle overpressure.

A third alternative is for a client to place a towel
behind their head and, holding the ends of the
towel, to use it to facilitate rotation themselves in
either supine or sitting position.

Mulligan (2010) says that by hooking the selvage
of the towel beneath the spinous process of a
specific vertebra and applying gentle force upward
and to one direction (e.g. right rotation or left
rotation) the client can help mobilize that
particular spinal segment. What do you think?

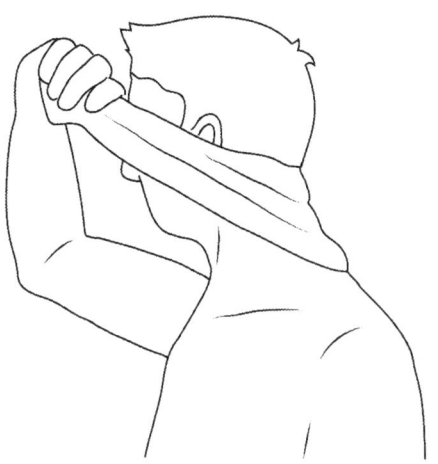

Mulligan, B.R., 2010. *Manual Therapy: NAGS, SNAGS, MWMS,*
etc. Plane View Services Ltd.

TIP 5 ENHANCING NECK STRETCHES

Many therapists are used to providing simple stretches as part of their homecare advice to clients. It is worth considering whether you could enhance the stretch by making minor alterations to the stretch position. In the case of lateral flexion, altering the position of the shoulder or altering the position of the head, or both, affects in which part of the neck the stretch is felt and, depending on the tension in those tissues, the intensity of the stretch.

Tip: One of the things to consider when teaching clients how to stretch their necks is that as they lengthen the muscles on one side of their necks they shorten muscles on the opposite side. This means that the shortened muscles sometimes cramp. Cramp is easily overcome by simply stetching out that side of the neck. However, if you know a client is prone to right-sided torticollis, for example, they should avoid stretching the left lateral flexors as doing so could trigger spasming of the muscles on the right side of their neck.

Here are some examples of how you could alter a simple lateral neck stretch to more specifically target the tense tissues:

a) Start with a simple lateral stretch in a neutral position. Take the head gently to the opposite side.

b) Retaining this position, actively depress the shoulder by pressing the elbow toward the floor.

c) Depress the shoulder by holding a chair prior to taking the head and neck into lateral flexion.

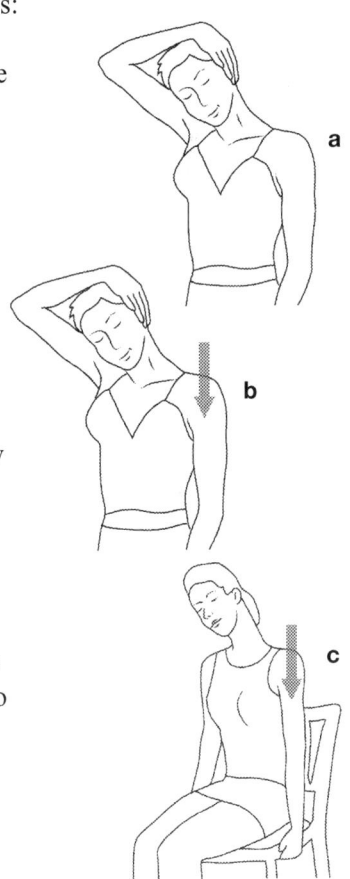

d) Hold a light weight (such as a bag of shopping) prior to taking the head and neck into lateral flexion.

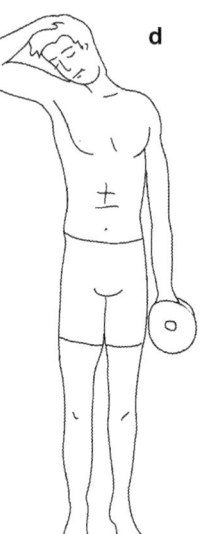

d

e) Resting in the supine position, depress the shoulder and fix the arm beneath the body prior to taking the neck into lateral flexion.

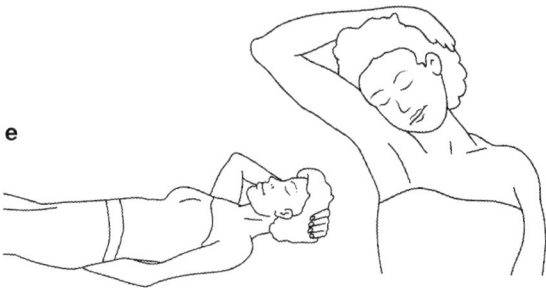

e

f) Alter the arm position: abduct the shoulder

g) Alter the arm: adduct the shoulder.

h) Alter the head position and notice how you can focus the stretch more to trapezius or more to levator scapulae. What position do you need to be in to move your head to get a better stretch of scalenes?

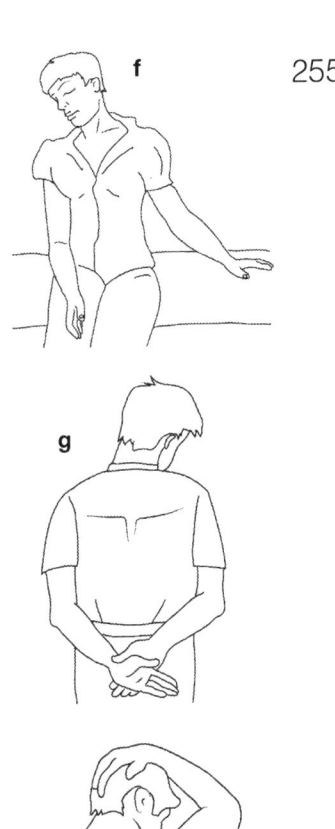

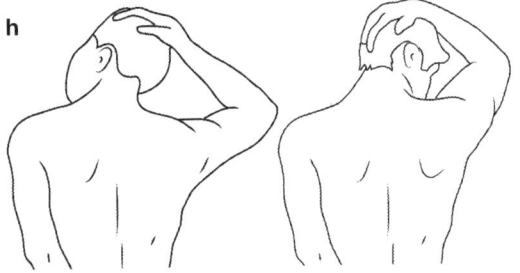

TIP 6 NECK ALIGNMENT WHILE SLEEPING

In *Part I, Tip* 9 (pp.52-53) you learned how you could draw around a client in order to get a better understanding of the distance between their head and shoulders.

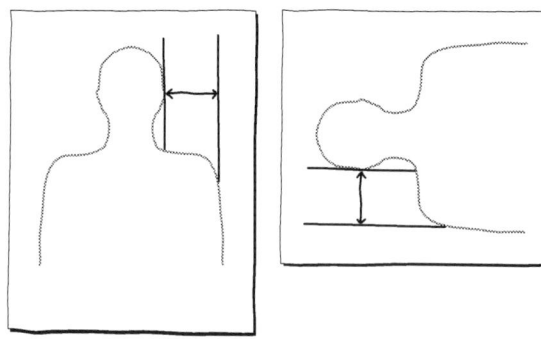

By turning this image on its side, through 90 degrees, you can use it to help explain to a client what happens to their neck when they rest on their side with too many (or too fat) pillows (**a**) and too few (or too thin) pillows (**b**). You can use this image to demonstrate how, when a person has a neck condition, such positions can aggravate the symptoms by either passively shortening the soft tissue on one side of the neck, in which case

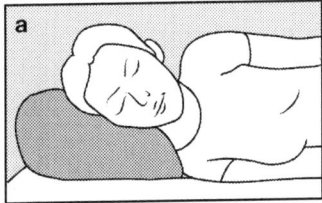

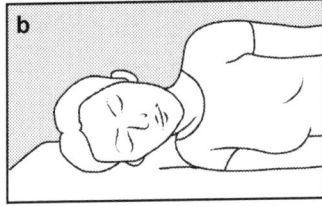

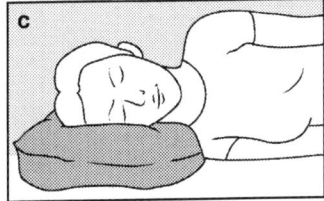

tissues on that side of the neck may cramp, while simultaneously lengthening the soft tissues on the other side of the neck, possibly overstretching them. Resting with the neck in lateral flexion in such a manner is not advisable. Using this same image from *Part I, Tip 9,* you can demonstrate to the client that correctly filling the gap between their shoulder and head (**c**) can help keep the cervical spine in a more neutral alignment, a position where tissues are neither shortened nor lengthened and cervical vertebrae can remain unstressed.

TIP 7 NECK RETRACTIONS

The center of gravity in humans falls slightly anterior to the transverse axis for flexion and extension of the head and neck. This means that our posterior neck muscles are active even when we are sitting or standing still, to prevent the head from falling forward. If you have ever seen anyone fall asleep on a train journey you might have noticed that their head tends to fall forward or to the side, as the posterior muscles relax and the weight of gravity pulls the head downward. They may jerk suddenly, as the cervical stretch reflex kicks in, when spindles in muscle fibers detect

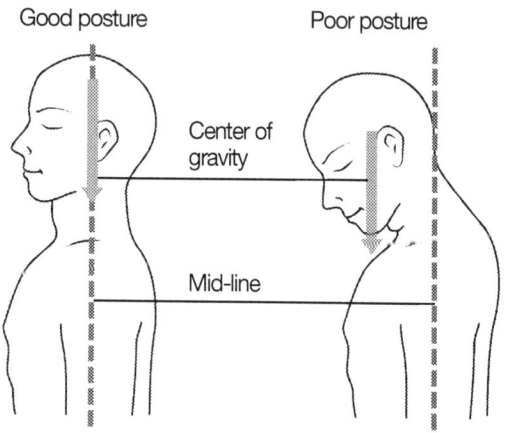

Good posture   Poor posture

Center of gravity

Mid-line

stretch and signal to the muscle group to contract.

When we maintain a static posture that involves looking down slightly, as when writing, reading a book or knitting, for example, our posterior neck muscles have to work hard to maintain our heads in this slightly flexed position, contracting eccentrically as we lower our heads into flexion, and concentrically to bring our heads back to the neutral position. They work even harder to bring about extension of the neck, as might be required when we look up to the ceiling when we are in the prone position. It is not suprising that many people experience tension and pain in their necks from the maintenance of static postures, and providing clients with an exercise they can do regularly to counteract this tension is highly beneficial. One such exercise is neck retraction.

This simple home care exercise is used to help clients with increased cervical lordosis and tension in the posterior neck muscles. It helps activate weakened deep neck flexors (longus coli and capitis). To perform neck retractions a client needs to give themselves a double chin by pulling their head backward. They could look in the mirror to observe their neck, or simply hold their hand on their chin as a guide.

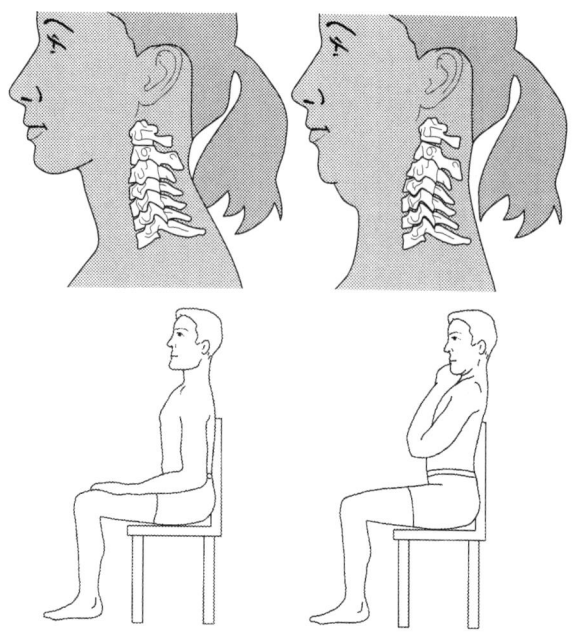

However, many clients find this difficult so it is

useful to practice first with them in supine on a treatment couch.

1. Place your finger in the mid point of their neck, touching their skin.
2. Ask the client to try and push their neck back into your finger.
3. As you feel them doing this, slowly move your finger toward the treatment couch, thus making the client retract their head and neck a little more.

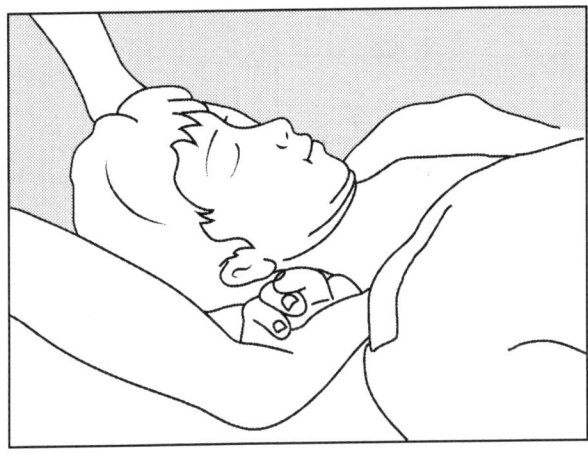

Use this exercise to explain the movement you need the client to perform while they are in a seated position.

In the seated position:

1. Suggest that the client imagines they have their chin resting on a shelf. This helps them keep their head facing forward. Without this command some clients extend their head and neck — a movement you want to avoid.

2. Note that it is important for the client to avoid sustained maximal contraction of muscles as they bring about retraction. Ask them to 'relax off' just a little so that they have changed the position of their head and neck yet are avoiding maximal contraction of scalenes.

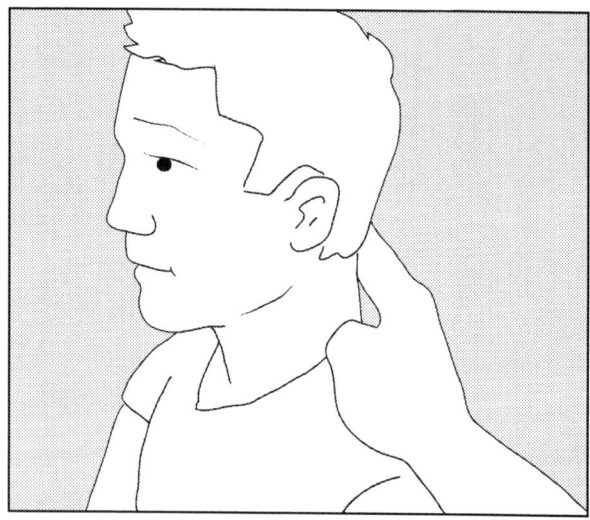

TIP 8 TRIGGER POINT MASSAGE

Using a spikey hard rubber or plastic therapy ball, clients can learn to treat trigger points all over their bodies, including the back of their necks where they can access the neck extensors.

Question: Are there any clients for whom self triggering is contraindicated?

Clients with acute conditions, such as osteoporosis, rheumatoid arthritis or another cervical condition that is contraindicated for massage, should avoid this treatment. Care should be taken by clients who bruise easily and all clients should be advised that they are aiming to reduce tension in the muscles of their necks, and so should avoid pressing hard onto the bones of their neck.

The table overleaf contrasts the advantages and disadvantages of using a therapy ball to deactivate trigger points in two different treatment positions—standing and supine.

Standing

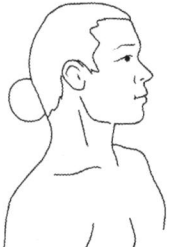

advantages	• This is a good starting point to experiment with how the client will respond to self management of trigger points, as the client can choose how much pressure they exert against the ball. • Is useful for when the client wants to use the ball during the day, at work for example. • The ball can be gently rolled up and down using simple nodding movement of the head, to access the suboccipital muscles.
disadvantages	• It can be difficult to keep the ball in place. • It requires pressing through muscles which are actively engaged in order to keep the head erect and may therefore decrease the effectiveness of accessing deeper muscles such as suboccipitals. • Some clients may find their quadriceps fatigue from having to make constant squatting movements as they maneuver the ball into place. • It can be difficult to move the ball left-to right. • If a client is particularly kyphotic or even just a little round-shouldered, it can be difficult getting close enough to the wall to access the back of the neck in this way.

Supine

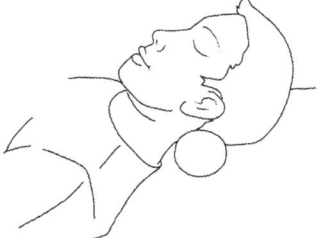

- The client can relax almost completely, letting their head roll side to side.
- This means that as tissues relax they may be able to access deeper soft tissue structures with the pressure of the ball.
- Some clients find it easier to access muscles to one side of their posterior neck in this way, as they can rest with their head in slight rotation.

- It can be difficult to access a trigger point above or below the point at which they are working as this means maneuvering themselves off the floor so that they can roll superior or inferior and onto the required trigger.
- The head is heavy and for some people there is a danger that this is too much pressure and they risk overtreating so good advice is to suggest that a client practices for a few minutes and see how their tissues respond the following day.

How to use a therapy ball to help deactivate trigger points

The illustrations on the next page show sites of common trigger points. Triggers are tender to touch and develop over many months or even years. Retention of a static upper body posture is thought to contribute to the development of trigger points in muscles of the neck. To treat these using a ball, gently press the ball onto the trigger point for about 30 seconds. The sensation should be slightly uncomfortable but not painful. Importantly, with gentle pressure this sensation should subside. When it subsides, press gently again into the point. Further discomfort should subside within about 60 seconds. Repeat about three times. Rub or massage the area following use of the ball. If the discomfort does not subside, do not apply further pressure. If, the following day, your neck feels sore or is bruised, you should not attempt trigger point work again. If, as is usually the case, your symptoms feel somewhat relieved, you can use the ball again, in the same manner.

Examples of common trigger points in the neck

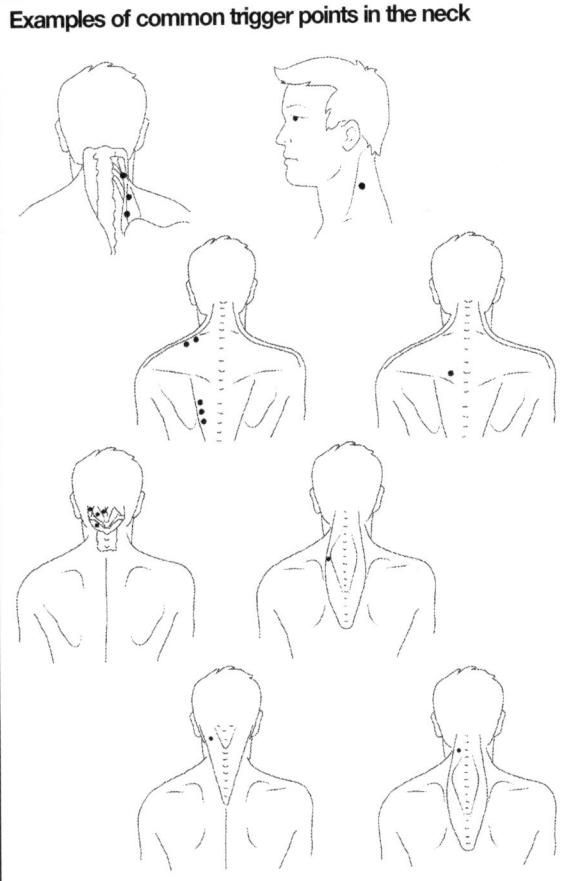

For further information see *The Trigger Point Therapy Workbook* by Claire Davies.

TIP 9 A TRICK WITH THE EYES!

This active technique improves cervical rotation.
Practice on yourself first to see how it works.

To increase rotation to the right

1. Turn your head to
the RIGHT as far as
you can.

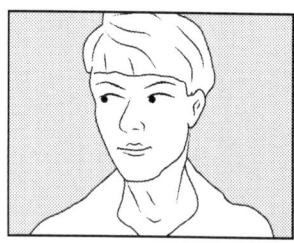

2. With your head in
this position move your
eyes as far as you can
to the LEFT. Hold for
10 seconds.

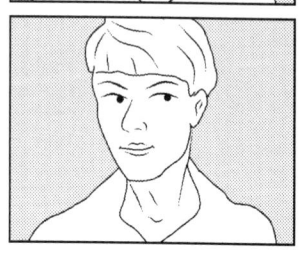

3. Now look RIGHT
and notice that you
gain a few millimeters
in right cervical
rotation.

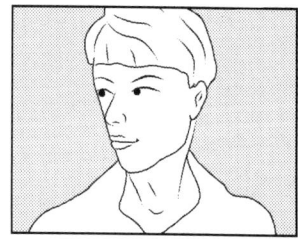

When teaching clients, remember to observe their cervical range of movement both before and after this activity.

To increase rotation to the left

1. Turn your head to the LEFT as far as you can.

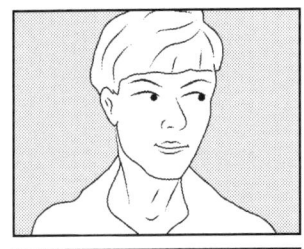

2. With your head in this position move your eyes as far as you can to the RIGHT. Hold for 10 seconds.

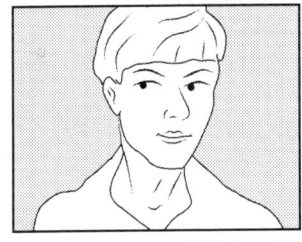

3. Now look LEFT and notice that you gain a few millimeters in left cervical rotation.

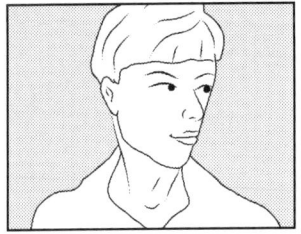

TIP 10   SELF MASSAGE

Using the examples shown here, teaching your client how to self massage their neck can be very helpful.

a Squeezing the occipital region
b Stroking or gripping neck extensors
c Using a theracane for trigger point work

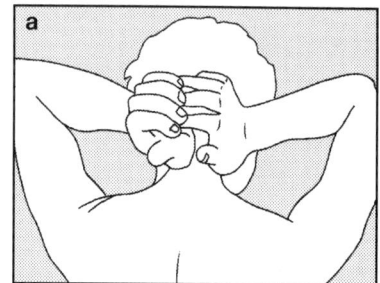

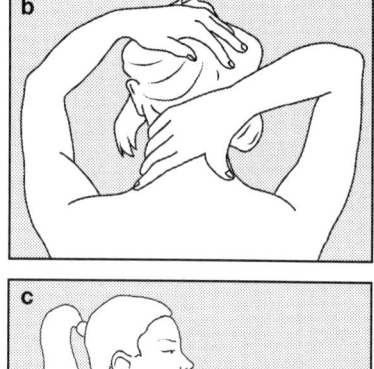

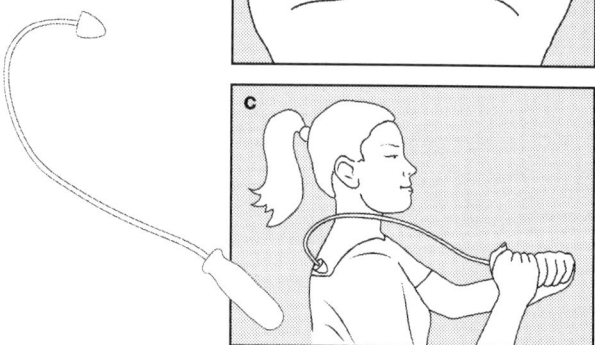

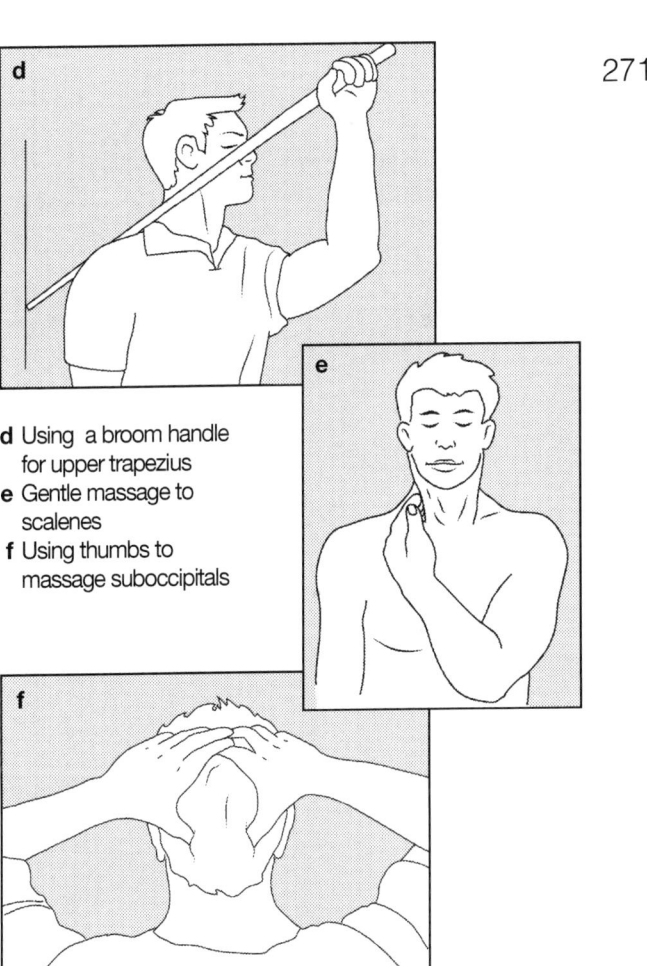

d Using a broom handle for upper trapezius
e Gentle massage to scalenes
f Using thumbs to massage suboccipitals

TIP 11 STRENGTHENING THE NECK

Isometric strengthening exercises are used for
strengthening weak muscles. Shown here are some

	Flexion	Extension	Right lateral flexion	
Isometric using hands				
Isometric using soft therapy ball				
Isometric strengthening using gravity				

of the simplest exercises. Isometric strengthening
can be done in these positions using bands, pulleys
and weights but are not shown here. Such
advanced isometric exercises and could cause
harm if performed without supervision.

Left lateral flexion	Right rotation	Left rotation

REFERENCES

Davies, C., *The Trigger Point Therapy Workbook*, 2004. Oakland, CA: New Harbinger.

Ezzo, J., Haraldsson B.G., Gross, A.R., Myers, C.D., Morien, A., Goldsmith, C.H., et al, 1976. Massage for mechanical neck disorders: a systematic review. *Spine* (Philadelphia, PA, 1976), 2007, 32:353-362.

Fairbanks, J.C., Couper, J., Davies, J.B., O'Brien, J.P., 1980. The Oswestry Low Back Pain Disability Questionnaire. *Physiotherapy*, 66:271-273.

Fallon, S. and Walsh, M., Positional Release Technique: a valid technique for use by physical therapy practitioners? IPTAS Conference (2012), Wordpress.com

Green, W.B., and Heckman, J.D, ed.,1993. *The Clinical Measurement of Joint Motion*. Rosemont, IL: American Academy of Orthopaedic Surgeons.

Hoving, J.L., O'Leary, E.F., Niere, K.R., Green, S., Buchbinder, R., 2003. Validity of the neck disability index, Northwick Park neck pain questionnaire, and problem elicitation technique for measuring disability associated with whiplash-associated disorders. *Pain*, 102(3):273-281

Johnson, J., *Postural Assessment*, 2012, Human Kinetics: Champaign, IL.

Johnson, J., *Soft Tissue Release*, 2009, Human Kinetics: Champaign, IL.

Leak, A.M., Cooper, J., Dyer, S., Williams, K.A., Turner-Stokes, L., Frank, A.O., 1994. The Northwick Park neck pain questionnaire, devised to measure neck pain and disability, 1994. *British Journal of Rheumatology,* 33:469-474.

Manheim, C.J. and Lavette, D.K., 1989. *The Myofascial Release Manual*. New Jersey: Slack Incorporated.

McPartland, J.M., Brodeur, R.R. and Hallgren, R.C., 1997. Chronic neck pain, standing balance, and suboccipital muscle atrophy — a pilot study. *Journal of Manipulative Physiological Therapeutics*, 20(1): 24-9.

Min, S.H., Chang, S-H., Jeon, S.K., Yoon, S.Z., Park, J-Y., and Shin, H.W., 2010. Posterior

276 auricular pain caused by the trigger points in the sternocleidomastoid muscle aggravated by psychological factors—a case report. *Korean Journal of Anaesthesiology*. 2010, Dec, 59 (Suppl): S229-S232.

Moseley, G.L., Impaired trunk muscle function in patients with sub-acute neck pain: etiologic in the subsequent development of low-back pain, 2004. *Manual Therapy*, 9:157-163.

Mulligan, B.R., 2010. *Manual Therapy: NAGS, SNAGS, MWMS, etc*. New Zealand: Plane View Services Ltd.

Ohashi, W., 1977. *Do-It-Yourself Shiatsu*. London: Unwin Paperbacks.

Sherman, K.J., Cherkin, D.C., Hawkes, R.J., Miglioretti, D.L., Deyo, R.A., 2009. Randomized trial of therapeutic massage for chronic neck pain. *Clinical Journal of Pain*, 25:233-238.

Shin, S., Yoon, D.M., York, K.B., 2011. Identification of the correct cervical level by palpation of spinous processes. *Anesth. Analog.* May 2011, 112(5):1232-5, Epub 2011 Feb 23

Vernon, H. and Mior, S., 1991. The Neck Disability Index: a study of reliability and validity. *Journal of Manipulative and Physiological Therapeutics*. 14, 409-415.

Wall, P., 1999. *Pain: The Science of Suffering*. London: Weidenfeld & Nicolson.

Watson, A.H.D., William C., and James, B.V., 2012. Activity Patterns in Latissiumus Dorsi and Sternocleidomastoid in Classical Singers. *J ournal of Voice*, 2012, May; 26(3):e95-e105